Fat Loss That Really work!

Balance Your Hormones:
- Insulin
- Estrogen
- Progesterone
- Testosterone
- Thyroid
- Cortisol
- DHEA

Look great!
Feel great!
Lose weight!
Have better sex!

Y.L. Wright, M.A.

Book Four in the Series,
"Bioidentical Hormones."

First Edition

Copyright © 2012 by Y.L. Wright, M.A.

All Rights Reserved. No part of this document may be reproduced without written consent from the author.

Published by Lulu.com in the United States

ISBN 978-1-105-24403-2

Printed in the United States of America

MEDICAL DISCLAIMER:

The following text is for general information only. It contains the opinions and ideas of the author. Careful attention has been paid to insure the accuracy of the information, but the author and the publisher cannot assume responsibility for the validity or consequences of its use. The intention of this book is to provide helpful information. This information is not intended to diagnose or treat any disease. This book is sold with the understanding that the author and publisher are not rendering medical, health, or any other professional services. See your medical or health professional concerning any health concerns or before following any suggestions made in this book or drawing inferences from it. The author and publisher specifically disclaim all responsibility for any liability, loss, or risk incurred as a direct or indirect consequence of using this book's contents. Any use of the information found in this book is the sole responsibility of the reader. Any dietary, nutrient, hormone, and medication suggestions found in this book are to be followed only under the supervision of a medical doctor or other endocrine specialist. Any reference to particular companies or supplements is only for the benefit of the reader. The author receives no compensation from endorsement of any product.

ACKNOWLEDGMENTS:

Back cover picture courtesy of Joe Swartz, MD. Thanks also to Dr. Swartz for editing this manuscript for medical accuracy.

Table of Contents

Introduction 5

Part I: Proven Weight Loss Methods 7

1.   Successful Weight Loss Methods for Many People 7

2.   Calorie Restriction..9
- *A.*   *Drink a shake and drop the fat...10*
- *B.*   *Some natural calorie restriction mimetics: 11*

3.   Exercise..12
- *A.*   *Strength training: 16*
- *B.*   *Flexibility training: 16*
- *C.*   *Aerobic endurance training: 16*
- *D.*   *Anaerobic training: 16*

4.   Other Successful Fat Loss Methods 17
- *A.*   *Is body sculpture (liposuction) safe and beneficial? 17*
- *B.*   *Weight loss surgery works for clinically severe and morbid obesity...........18*
- *C.*   *Pharmaceuticals may help with fat loss. 18*
- *D.*   *Other substances to lose fat include: 19*

5.   To Lose Fat in the Long Run, Remember:................................20

6.   Many People Can't Lose Weight! 21
- *A.*   *Why most diets fail. 21*
- *B.*   *Poor lifestyle habits lead to weight gain...................................22*

Part II: Balance Hormones: Lose Fat 24

7.   Most Overweight People Have Hormone Imbalances! 24

8.   Improve Digestion for Hormone Health..................................25

9.   Too Much Insulin...26
- *A.*   *Metabolic syndrome is a major cause and result of obesity. 26*
- *B.*   *This is what happens when you have insulin resistance...............27*
- *C.*   *Insulin resistance leads to diabetes, cancer, heart disease. 28*
- *D.*   *Let's prevent/reduce insulin resistance.....................................29*

10.   Control Carbohydrates 30
- *A.*   *Eat the right amount of carbohydrate. 30*

4 Fat Loss Secrets that Really Work!

B.	Eat the right kind of carbs.	30
C.	Check your carbohydrate metabolism.	31
D.	Avoid artificial sweeteners.	32
E.	Alcohol harms us in many ways.	32
F.	Low-carb diets are harmful over time.	32

11. Low-Fat Diets Impair Hormones and Health. 33

12. *Balance* Your Diet for Hormone Health 35

13. Estrogen Dominance 37

A.	Excess belly fat makes us get even fatter.	37
B.	Fat-soluble toxins are stored in fat, especially belly fat.	38
C.	Foods to cleanse metabolic wastes:	38
D.	Obese people have high estrogen in relation to the other hormones.	39
E.	Artificial estrogens make us fat.	40
F.	Symptoms of estrogen dominance:	41
G.	How to treat estrogen dominance.	42

14. Heal the Adrenals, Then the Thyroid 45

A.	Cortisol is a stress hormone produced by the adrenals.	45
B.	Progesterone drops with stress	47
C.	Stress drops men's testosterone.	47
D.	To balance your hormones, control stress.	48
E.	DHEA declines with stress, aging, and weight gain.	49

15. An Underactive Thyroid 50

A.	Don't eat a low carb diet.	51
B.	Take the right amount of iodine.	51
C.	Get an accurate diagnosis and treatment.	51
D.	If you have a lot of Reverse T3,	53
E.	Get a physical to check your thyroid.	53
F.	If you have anti-thyroid antibodies, be sure to try a gluten-free diet.	53
G.	Low thyroid is associated with impaired digestion.	53

Part III: Flying into Action 54

16. Find a Physician Who Will Treat All Hormone Imbalances 54

17. Treatment Plan to Balance Hormones 55

INDEX 57

REFERENCES 58

Introduction

BEING OVERWEIGHT CAUSES HEALTH ISSUES THAT MAY KILL YOU. If you don't want to die younger, normalize your weight. If you are 50 years old and obese, you are shortening the rest of your life by two or three times. [1]

Read this book and learn how to implement strategies into your lifestyle that have been PROVEN to be successful in losing fat and keeping it off permanently. You will learn how *everyone* can be successful long-term with achieving fat loss. This book looks at what has actually worked for people to lose weight for the rest of their lives. You will learn how to structure your lifestyle to lose the fat and keep it off permanently, without resorting to one of the latest diet fads.

Many people wait for the next best-selling diet book to come out and tell them how to lose weight. But these popular weight loss methods and diets do not work long-term and may be dangerous to your health when followed for any length of time.[2] Research shows that the vast majority of people using these diets will slowly gain the weight back.[3]

Perhaps you have tried many of the weight-loss programs out there. You lost weight for a while, but didn't have long-term success. You tried the diets, the gyms, the personal trainers, the weight-loss centers—but still your weight keeps going up as the years roll by.

The problem is that none of these methods have looked at your hormones. Hormonal balance is critical if you want to lose fat and keep it off. Few people understand the importance of hormonal balance in maintaining proper weight. Fewer still understand how to achieve hormonal balance.

When you go to a weight loss center or a gym, hormones are usually not addressed. Until you address your hormonal issues, you will not achieve long-term success with your attempts at weight loss.

6 Fat Loss Secrets that Really Work!

Most overweight people have unbalanced hormones, more so if they have been dieting on and off for years and years. The process of repetitive dieting does the same thing to your hormones that is caused by the aging process. Read this book and learn how your hormones change with dieting and aging and exactly what you can do to get back into balance. Find out which hormones become unbalanced through dieting and specifically how to bring them back into balance so that you can normalize your weight and improve your health.

Learn exactly how to correct the hormonal problems that prevent you from losing fat, especially belly fat, and how to finally normalize your weight for life. You will be given the information you need to finally lose the excess pounds that you have been lugging around all these years.

This book is the fourth book in the series, "Bioidentical Hormones." My mission in writing these books is to bring you the latest scientific information gleaned from hundreds of lectures given by anti-aging physicians and supported by research presented in medical journals. Read the other books in the "Bioidentical Hormones" series:

1. Secrets about Bioidentical Hormones to Lose Fat and Prevent Cancer, Heart Disease, Menopause, and Andropause by Optimizing Adrenals, Thyroid, Estrogen, Progesterone, Testosterone, and Growth Hormone!

2. Bioidentical Hormones Made Easy!

3. Secrets About Growth Hormone to Build Muscle, Increase Bone Density, and Burn Body Fat!

5. Secrets about the HCG Diet! Treatment Guide, Controversy, Benefits, Risks, Side Effects, and Contraindications.

All of my books can be purchased in either print or downloadable versions at: http://www.lulu.com/spotlight/treewise

Part I: Proven Weight Loss Methods

We will look first at the weight-loss methods that have been proven to be successful for many people. Then we will see why these methods don't work for everyone and find strategies that WILL work for everyone.

1. Successful Weight Loss Methods for Many People

THE POPULAR DIETS DON'T WORK IN THE LONG-TERM. Most people don't lose a *significant* amount of weight in the long-term on any of the best-selling diets. Not Atkins, Ornish, Weight Watchers, or Zone, not any of them. People typically lose weight initially, but ultimately the weight comes back . . . and with a vengeance.

Most people that followed any of these diets lost only 2-3% of their body weight. This is not metabolically significant. The diets are difficult to maintain for long periods of time and do not produce a metabolically significant amount of weight loss.[4]

Eating high or low protein doesn't matter when it comes to long-term weight loss. The differences in these popular diets revolve around amounts of protein, carbohydrates, and fats. But the research shows that effective weight loss doesn't revolve around the amount of calories coming from protein, carbohydrates, and fat. The newest guidelines from the Institute of Medicine, Food and Nutrition Board[5] have wide ranges for each of these nutrients.

The only diet that works to lose weight in the long-term is calorie restriction. Caloric restriction is one of the few things proven to prolong longevity.

8   Fat Loss Secrets that Really Work!

People can choose to eat low protein or high protein, low carbohydrate or high carbohydrate, low fat or high fat. In terms of long-term weight loss, it doesn't really matter. The only diet that works for people in the long-term is calorie restriction.

Percentage of calories from proteins, carbohydrates, and fats does matter in other aspects of health, which we will discuss later, but not in weight loss. We will go into detail later about how to *balance* your diet and make healthy food choices to insure your health.

The people who do lose a significant amount of weight and keep it off do two things: [6]

1) They restrict the amount of calories that they eat.
2) They exercise for a half hour or more every day.

The largest group who has been successful at losing weight and keeping it off long-term is the National Weight Control Registry.[7] To qualify for this group, you must have lost about thirty pounds and kept it off for five years. Not many people qualify. The few who do are registered into the group by their physicians.

This is what the people in this group have done to lose the fat and keep it off for at least five years:

1) 98% of Registry participants modified their food intake in some way to lose weight.
2) 94% increased their physical activity, with the most frequently reported form of activity being walking.[8]

Let's look first at calorie restriction and exercise, the two proven methods of losing weight. Then we will
look at the other methods that have been shown to work. Finally and most importantly, we will see why many people *can't* lose weight because of hormonal imbalances caused by environmental pollution, pharmaceuticals, altered food supply, poor eating habits, and improper lifestyle.

Read on and learn the secrets that will allow you to overcome all health obstacles, achieve hormonal balance, and finally lose all of your unwanted fat and keep it off forever! Follow these tips to look great, feel great, lose weight and have better sex!

2. Calorie Restriction

WHEN YOU RESTRICT CALORIES, YOU WILL LIVE A LONGER LIFE. Calorie restriction causes many favorable changes in your body. Okinawan centenarians practice a cultural calorie control habit called "hara hachi bu." They eat until they are only 80% full. For those of us who can do this, the health benefits are many.

Positive effects of calorie restriction include:
- Reduction in heart rate.
- Reduction in body fat, especially belly fat.
- Improvements in cardiovascular structure and function.
- Reduction in blood pressure.[9]
- Reduction in LDL cholesterol.
- Reduction in triglycerides.
- Improvements in insulin sensitivity and blood glucose levels.
- Increase in protein synthesis and elimination of abnormal proteins.
- Improvement in the repair and maintenance of cells.
- Reduction of oxidative stress by decrease in free radical formation.
- Increase in muscle mass.
- Better production of hormones that fall with age (HGH and DHEA).
- Improvements in brain function, including memory, cognition, and mood.
- Increased ability to exercise.
- Stimulation of growth factors.
- Decrease in inflammation.
- Weight loss.

Unfortunately, not many of us have that kind of self-control. Not even many Okinawans practice calorie restriction these days. This way of eating is dying off with the advent of fast-food restaurants. As Okinawans adopt the American way of eating, many have now become overweight. This is a shame, because the Okinawan way of eating is quite healthy. Their diet is rich in natural anti-oxidants, Omega-3 fatty acids, and minerals. This is a low-calorie, yet nutrient-dense diet.

This is the diet that has been found by anti-aging researchers to offer life extension benefits. This diet is the exact opposite of the typical diet found in most modern societies.

Americans are eating more and more. Statistics show that both men and women are eating more calories each day as time goes on. Calorie intake has gone up drastically in the last four decades. Overweight and obesity have risen proportionately from consuming the Standard American Diet (S.A.D.).[10]

You really do need to cut down your calorie intake if you want to lose fat. Cut down portion size. Cut down boredom eating. Stop snacking on junk food. Cut down calories.

A. Drink a shake and drop the fat. There is good
data to show that substituting a low-calorie diet formula (a shake) for one meal a day will help you drop the fat. Researchers in Spain found a startling difference in weight loss between a group using diet alone and a group using diet with a shake as a meal replacement. They concluded that, "Substitution of a low-calorie diet formula for a meal is an effective measure for weight loss maintenance compared with dieting alone."[11] Drink the shake for breakfast and a healthy 200-calorie snack bar or low-glycemic snack in the afternoon. This is an easy way to cut down your calories.

Some foods and supplements mimic the good effects of calorie restriction and help you lose fat. [12] The good news is that we can still get many of the benefits of calorie restriction *without* restricting calories. If you can't develop the self-control to limit your calorie intake, there are now products that you can take that will give you many of the same benefits of calorie restriction.

A calorie restriction mimetic is a pharmaceutical, chemical compound, or natural agent that can mimic the benefits of calorie restriction. Calorie restriction mimetics often regulate blood glucose and decrease insulin resistance. This makes it easier to lose weight. They may be taken along with calorie restriction for even greater health benefits.

B. Some natural calorie restriction mimetics:

- ***Resveratrol.*** This key anti-aging agent has proven anti-cancer and cardiovascular benefits. It is a potent anti-oxidant.
- ***Cinnamon.*** It acts like insulin.
- ***Carnosine.*** It inhibits the formation of toxic sugar residues (glycosylated end products) which result from eating excessive sugar loads and which produce metabolic syndrome and type 2 diabetes.
- ***Ellagic Acid.*** It is in raspberries and pomegranates and has a potent anti-cancer effect.
- ***Grape seed extract.*** Anti-cancer, good for the heart.
- ***Green tea.*** Anti-cancer, good for the heart. Increases the liver's ability to burn fat.
- ***Maritime pine bark.*** Anti-cancer, good for the heart.
- ***Avocado.*** Increases insulin sensitivity.
- ***Chromium.*** Modulates sugar metabolism and increases insulin sensitivity.
- ***Vanadium.*** Modulates sugar metabolism.
- ***Alpha-Lipoic Acid.*** An insulin sensitizer and antioxidant.
- ***Gymnema alkaloids.*** Found in Ayurvedic Medicine.
- ***Sleep.*** Getting plenty of sleep may help people to lose weight even though they do nothing else to lose weight!
- ***Acetyl-L-Carnitine.*** Facilitates mitochondrial function.
- ***Leptin.*** Stimulates fat metabolism.

Metformin is an anti-diabetic drug that increases insulin sensitivity and modulates stress responses.

Although it is a drug, it is invaluable when used to get control of abnormal blood sugar. It is very helpful for the obese, type 2 diabetic to prevent further destruction of the pancreas and allow healing. Some anti-diabetic drugs stimulate the pancreas to produce more insulin. These increase pancreatic burn-out, leading to greatly increased diabetes in the long run.

3. Exercise

HOW DOES THE RIGHT AMOUNT OF EXERCISE HELP US TO LOSE WEIGHT? To lose weight you need to burn more energy than you take in. Can you walk? If the answer is yes, do it. Build up to an hour or more of walking each day. Pedometers are motivating for some people, as they can add up all of the walking they do during the whole day. By spreading out the walking over the course of the day, the walking really adds up. If you walk for a half hour three times a day, you will actually burn more calories than you would if you walk for an hour and a half once a day. When you bump up your metabolism more frequently, it *stays* up so that you burn more calories even when you aren't exercising. If you can't walk, find something you *can* do like riding a stationary bike. If you have knee/leg pain that limits walking, exercise in water. Join a gym and go. Just do it.

Even if you are really obese, you can exercise and gain huge benefits. Forget about the amount of weight you need to lose. First concentrate on getting healthier. When you can burn 3000 calories a week at a moderately-intense level of activity (not working out all *that* hard) you will see improvement in every health-care marker that exists. This includes triglycerides, blood pressure, body composition, HDL, and blood glucose tolerance. Exercise is the cure for diabetes, if it's type 2 and caught early.[13]

You will see improvement in every health marker immediately, even after the very first exercise session.[14] You will continue to improve with every exercise session. You will be able to return to the natural state of health that your body was designed for. You will sleep better. Disease will melt away as you keep at it. Your sex life will improve. There is no drug that can do what exercise will do.

Now that you have started exercising, let me let you in on a little secret that will really help you to lose that fat and gain the muscle that is needed to keep the fat off. It is called anaerobic training.

Anaerobic training is important for all people at any age. In order to keep muscle on your body, do some type of anaerobic training. It involves working out so hard that you must slow down, stop to catch your breath, or stop and let your muscles recover in between sets. Types of anaerobic activity include weight lifting, interval training, martial arts, and sprinting.

The more intense the activity, the better it is, unless you have disease: heart disease, inflammatory illnesses, chronic pain, chronic fatigue syndrome, etc. Not only will you burn more calories, but you will help your endocrine system to work better to keep your hormone levels balanced, especially as you age.[15]

High-intensity exercise will help all of your endocrine glands to work better than any other type of exercise. If you are a walker or a jogger, try some sprinting. Go as fast as you can for short distances. It may seem hard at first, but you can do it if you are relatively healthy, no matter how old or out of shape you are. Just start out with a few brief easy sprints and work up to doing more and more.

Get your heart rate up high enough so that you move up out of the fat burning zone (60%-70% of your maximum heart rate for age) and into the heart strengthening zone. Your maximum heart rate is found by subtracting your age from 220. You will lose more fat doing this than you will if you stay in that classical fat burning zone.[16]

You can find out your heart rate by riding stationary bikes or treadmills or other exercise equipment that shows you your heart rate. Or you can get a heart rate monitor. Or you can look at your watch and take your pulse for six seconds and multiply by ten.

When you gain muscle as well as lose fat, you will look great. Muscle is your secret fat-burning machine. If you only lose fat, the skin just hangs on you. Looking like a concentration camp survivor is not healthy. To get healthy you need to lose fat and gain muscle. You need to improve your body composition. Then you will really look good in your swimsuit. Muscle gives you the sexy contours that make you look attractive. You can gain muscle by doing strength training.

Don't rely on the scale. Look in the mirror. Muscle is heavier than fat. When you gain muscle while losing fat, you will weigh more according to the scale. This is OK. Building muscle tissue is healthy. The more muscle tissue you have, the higher your metabolism. More muscle makes you burn more fat. The mirror will show your real progress. The scale may say that you have gained weight, but in the mirror you can see that you are looking great as you lose the fat and gain the muscle.

In order to improve body composition you must increase muscle and lose fat. Body composition is far-improved when strength training is combined with aerobic training. This decreases risk for diseases, including metabolic syndrome.[17]

Combine strength training with cardio training for best results. When strength training is combined with aerobic training, fat loss triples and muscle is gained.[18]

Exercise which targets the burning of belly fat is important. Compared to fat found in the upper legs and buttocks, visceral fat (belly fat) is much more strongly linked to cardiovascular disease and diabetes.[19] Certainly any aerobic exercise will help you lose the belly fat. But it is also important to add in specific abdominal exercises such as Pilates and other core exercise to lose the dangerous abdominal fat.

Motivation is tough, but you can do it. For many people, it is tough to get going with an exercise program. They go to the doctor and expect a pill to take care of their weight problems. But no pill can take the place of physical activity. You just have to do it.

If you don't have the willpower to get going with an exercise program, find someone to exercise with. If you have a friend who will walk with you, then get together and always exercise at a certain time of each day. Get a dog. You *have to* walk the dog. Join a gym and get a personal trainer to design a program for you. Get a work-out partner to share in the fun.

Years ago, people didn't have to worry about finding the time and motivation to exercise. Exercise was a part of everyday life. My grandfather used to walk ten miles a day to work on a farm doing heavy labor. He didn't need to go to the gym. Rates of heart disease, cancer, obesity, and diabetes were extremely low a hundred years ago.

Now we have cars that take us to the supermarket. We sit in front of our computers and televisions. Our technological marvels make life so easy. But if we want to enjoy health, we must make a daily effort to exercise and eat properly. Before you go to the doctor for a pill to take care of your ills, exercise and eat properly. If everyone did this, we would see a reversal in most of the chronic illnesses that we see today.

Excuses for not exercising just don't cut it. Devise strategies to overcome your excuses. Figure out how to get over your excuses and just do it. A popular excuse is, "I can't go to the gym until I lose some weight because I look terrible." Fears about what other people in the gym are thinking about you are unfounded in reality. The gym is actually very motivating because everybody there is also working out. When I see overweight people in the gym, I smile at them and give them respect for showing up. I always think, "Good for them. I hope they keep it up!" You just have to show up and do it.

The bottom line on exercise is to do it and keep doing it for the rest of your life. The American College of Sports Medicine (ACSM) sums it up, "Emphasis should be placed on factors that result in permanent lifestyle change and encourage a lifetime of physical activity." [20]

The ACSM tells you to do it and do it all to keep fit and healthy. "A well-rounded training program including aerobic and resistance training and flexibility exercises is recommended." A good work-out starts with a warm-up, then strength training, some endurance training, some sprinting, and some flexibility exercises at the end when your muscles are loose. There you have it.

But don't overdo. Excessive exercise can cause weight gain by harming your adrenals. It will cause too much cortisol (a stress hormone) to be produced. The cortisol causes fat to be stored,[21] pushing your adrenals into adrenal fatigue or exhaustion. Excessive exercise also produces free radicals which cause inflammation. Don't forget to take antioxidants to handle free radical production. For most people, a rule of thumb is, "Don't exercise for more than two hours a day to avoid excessive cortisol production, resulting fat storage, and adrenal burn-out."

To become healthy, lose unwanted fat and gain muscle, include these types of training:

A. Strength training: *Consult an exercise professional to show you how to isolate each muscle group and train properly.* Start easy and gradually make your work-outs harder to avoid injury. Stimulate the body hard enough so that it will build muscle to adapt to the change. Begin by finding a weight that you can lift at least 8 times but not more than 15 times in each set. When you can lift it more than 15 times, add some weight. Make sure that in each set you push your muscles all the way to the point where you can't do another rep. Don't rest in between reps. Wait until the set is done. Then rest long enough so that you can lift the weight as many times as you did in the first set. Do 3-6 sets. If you are taking Growth Hormone or Testosterone, you will gain much more muscle with strength training. Hormone replacement therapy is much less effective without strength training. For more information on replacing these hormones, please read Book One[22] and Book Three[23] in the Bioidentical Hormone series.

B. Flexibility training: Stretch at least three times a week. Don't stretch past pain. This will make your muscles tighten up, and you risk injury. Hold the stretch for 30-60 seconds or until the muscle releases and you deepen into the stretch, and then stretch a bit further.

C. Aerobic endurance training: Jog, walk, ride a bike, or get on the cardio equipment four times a week up to every day. Start with low intensity for ten minutes and gradually build it up to an hour. Keep going at a rate that you can hang onto without having to stop and rest.

D. Anaerobic training: If healthy, start with two sprint sessions of 15-30 seconds of sprinting twice a week. Add another sprint session with each work-out until you get up to at least eight sprint sessions. Give yourself a four minute recovery time in between the sprints. During the recovery time, just move slowly to prevent lactic acid from building up in your muscles. Reduce the recovery time to two minutes as you become more fit. Swim if you can't run, and do sprints in the water.

4. Other Successful Fat Loss Methods

***CALORIE RESTRICTION AND EXERCISE* work for many people to keep the weight off long-term.** We have discussed the specifics of each and exactly how to implement them into our lifestyle. Now let's look at the other methods that have been used by people to successfully lose fat and keep it off.

A. Is body sculpture (liposuction) safe and beneficial?[24]

Targeted liposuction of up to four liters of fat from the subcutaneous tissue compartment:

- Improves insulin resistance.
- Lowers LDL cholesterol and triglycerides.
- Reduces C-reactive protein (a marker for inflammation).
- Reduces appetite.
- Facilitates weight management over time.

Caution must be advised when choosing to do liposuction.[25] It requires anesthesia, and death is a possible complication of anesthesia. Liposuction doesn't change your lifestyle and what put the fat there in the first place. Concerns are for complications like hemorrhage, infection, and creating scar tissue in the areas of liposuction.

Contraindications to liposuction include:

- Having been on Accutane less than 6 months prior to the procedure.
- Connective tissue disorders.
- Significant stretch marks.
- Blood clotting disorders.
- Lupus.
- Diabetes.
- Heart or lung disease.
- Vascular problems (including common circulation problems).
- Endocrine disorders.
- Hypertension.
- Depression.
- Other active diseases may affect outcome or increase risks.

18   Fat Loss Secrets that Really Work!

- Morbid obesity.
- Wound healing disorders.
- Smoking.
- Recreational drug use or excessive drinking.
- Pregnancy.

B. Weight loss surgery works for clinically severe and morbid obesity. Morbid obesity is having a body mass index (BMI) greater than or equal to 35. Weight loss surgery works for certain patients when less-invasive methods of weight loss have failed.[26] These patients are at great risk for numerous diseases that lead to death.

The use of weight loss surgery has increased dramatically recently.[27] Bariatric surgeons can do gastric bypass, gastric banding, and they are creating new surgical interventions to aid in fat loss.

Patients who are at risk for obesity-related morbidity or mortality (diseases and death caused by obesity) may qualify for gastric bypass surgery. This involves greatly reducing the size of the stomach. This option is a last resort, as it is risky.

Consider all other options before resorting to surgery, especially when treating children. Your chances of a successful outcome improve when you choose a surgeon that specializes in this type of surgery and does many of these procedures each week. Average hospital stay is down to three days. If you have co-morbidities or are twice your ideal body weight, insurance will often pay for this surgery.

C. Pharmaceuticals may help with fat loss.

But they are not as powerful as the above strategies and come with their own set of side effects.

D. Other substances to lose fat include:

- ***Chromium picolinate.***[28]
- ***Decaffeinated green coffee.***[29]
- ***Phaseolus vulgaris*** (a white bean extract).[30] It slows carbohydrate metabolism. Take once or twice a day with meals. Obese adults will lose abdominal fat and reduce triglyceride levels.
- ***Hydroxy citric acid.***[31] The FDA has issued a warning about the use of "Hydroxycut." It works by reducing hunger.
- ***Green tea.*** Catechin antioxidants in green tea reduce body fat and help control obesity. Green tea combats insulin resistance.[32] Products vary widely in green tea amounts, so read the labels.
- ***Vanadyl sulfate*** taken with meals will mimic insulin.[33]
- ***Fucoxanthins with pomegranate seed oil*** increase metabolic rate, and induce fat burning.[34]
- ***7 Keto DHEA*** in the morning and at lunch. It drives liver cells to burn fatty acids for energy, lowering triglycerides in the liver.
- ***Irvingia*** twice a day with food helps to control appetite.[35] [36] To avoid yo-yo dieting, continue a maintenance dose so that the brain does not register hunger,
- ***Tryptophan*** is an amino acid that converts into serotonin. It should be taken at bedtime. Supplementation has been effectively used for sleep disorders, depression, and eating disorders.[37] Tryptophan enhances the release of serotonin from neurons in the brain. This decreases appetite for carbohydrates. When fewer carbs are eaten, people lose weight.[38] Raising tryptophan levels may decrease cravings and binge eating.[39]
- ***Non-stimulant appetite suppressants***—Hoodia gordonii, Caralluma fimbriata, increased fiber.
- ***Thermogenic agents***—Increased body heat helps to burn fat. These include citrus aurantium, fucoxanthins, natural amines (p-synephrine), and green tea.

5. To Lose Fat in the Long Run, Remember:

- **_NO SUPPLEMENT ALONE_ will make you lose fat permanently. You must reduce calories and eat a healthy diet.**

- **Pharmaceuticals (both over-the-counter and prescription) may have toxic side effects.**

- **Reducing 500 calories a day will help you to lose 1-2 pounds a week. This is a healthy rate of weight loss.**

- **Lose 1-2 pounds a week to keep the weight off.**

- **Exercise for at least thirty minutes a day. Walking is good. Find something you like and stick with it.**

- **Psychological counseling sometimes helps.**

- **Nutritional counseling helps when you hit a plateau.**

- **Even a modest fat loss will improve your health dramatically**. If you are fifty pounds overweight, you don't have to lose all fifty pounds to improve your health significantly. Even a modest 7-15% loss of excess fat will produce profound changes in your health. It will reduce your risk of dying early and will improve all of your other health parameters. It's OK to take baby steps.

Let's see why diet and exercise may not be the only answer and how these methods may actually be counter-productive to weight loss in some people. Let's look next at what we can do when the usual weight loss methods of calorie restriction and exercise haven't been working, and we don't want to resort to surgery or pills.

6. Many People Can't Lose Weight!

61% OF ALL AMERICANS ARE OVERWEIGHT!

That's over 160 million people. Almost a third of the population is classified as obese![40] We all know that exercise and good nutrition helps us to lose weight. Most people can control these factors if they have the willpower. But willpower alone isn't enough to control what happens to our bodies as we age or as we gain and lose weight. What can a person do to lose weight rather than just trying to find an optimal diet to attempt to correct the problem? Read on.

A. Why most diets fail.

Most people lose weight, but then gain it back, lose it again, and then gain it back again. Most diets fail because when people lose weight by dieting, they lose not only fat, but also lean muscle. This results in a decrease in metabolism which causes excessive weight gain over the long-term. Diets may injure metabolism, making future attempts to decrease weight futile. You cannot lose weight with diseased or bad metabolism.

The problem with yo-yo dieting is that the more people diet, the more difficult it becomes to lose weight. Roller coaster dieting causes us to lose lean muscle which decreases our metabolism. When metabolism decreases, it becomes harder and harder to keep the fat off. Most people who go on diets tend to regain the weight . . . and more.

Diets that cause slow metabolism and muscle loss are counter-productive. They include starvation and ketosis diets for long periods of time, very low calorie diets (less than 800 calories a day), long-term use of appetite suppressants, and eating less than three meals a day. When you don't eat often enough, your body stores the food as fat, because it knows it won't get fed again soon enough. These diets can produce Wilson's Temperature Syndrome and precipitate a change in the peripheral conversion of thyroid hormone. This not only dramatically slows metabolism and increases weight, but lowers energy, depresses mood, slows thinking, and decreases detoxification and cleansing of the

22   Fat Loss Secrets that Really Work!

body. It can be hard to diagnose because the thyroid blood tests are normal (TSH).

On crash diets, the body thinks it is starving and begins to hibernate to survive. When calories are reduced, the body thinks it is starving and slows down the conversion of the inactive thyroid hormone, T4, to the active thyroid hormone, T3, which can be used by our cells to make energy. Essentially, you go into hibernation, like a bear in winter. This protected mankind against famine and winters without food for thousands of years. You slow down the fat burning, so you can make it through the winter when there is not enough food to the spring when you can get enough food again.

Caution is advised for obese people who go on crash diets. When calorie intake is drastically restricted, the effects on obese people are actually counterproductive. Drastic calorie reduction can turn down the metabolic rate in several ways:

1.   Decreasing muscle mass produces decreased metabolism of calories.
2.   It may produce Wilson's syndrome and hypothyroidism.[41]
3.   It may harm the adrenals and produce adrenal dysfunction, even resulting in decreased sex hormones.
4.   It may increase the release of harmful toxins, which may increase insulin resistance.
5.   Bone density also decreases with very low calorie diets.[42]
6.   Gallstone formation increases.[43]
7.   Uric acid levels increase which may lead to gout.[44]

On crash diets, water and muscle are lost faster than fat, and it becomes harder to burn fat. Obese people who *really* want to try a very low calorie diet may want to consider going on the hCG protocol, because the hCG helps to burn that unwanted fat around your thighs, belly, and the back of your arms, while maintaining muscle mass. See book five in the "Bioidentical Hormone" series, <u>Secrets about the HCG Diet!</u> [45]

B. Poor lifestyle habits lead to weight gain.

- Most people don't eat properly. Most Americans are following diets that are nutrient-poor and filled with toxins.
- Many don't exercise, or if they do, they don't continue on with regular exercise.

Fat Loss Secrets that Really Work! 23

- They have poor sleep hygiene (bad sleep habits).
- They eat fast food (nutrient-poor and filled with toxins).
- They eat empty calories, which are nutrient-poor and processed to death.
- People who skip breakfast are 450 times more likely to be overweight and obese. If we let ourselves get hungry, we tend to eat too much in one meal. Eating too much in one meal slows down metabolism.

Other factors in weight gain include:
- Many people have diseases.
- Medications may affect weight gain and weight loss.
- Genetics cause many people to become fatter than others.
- Emotional issues play a big part. Depressed people eat to nurture themselves. Anxious people eat to calm themselves. People may armor themselves with fat to avoid the attentions of the opposite sex. The stress hormone, cortisol, plays a big role in weight gain. Stress, anxiety, and depression all elevate cortisol, until the adrenals burn out. Eventually these emotional issues may result in adrenal fatigue and adrenal exhaustion. Do everything you can to stop the chronic stress. Turn off the cell phone, turn off the TV, and meditate on your breath.
- Diseases create fat, usually by destroying the metabolism.

To normalize your weight, exercise regularly and:
- Balance your diet with plenty of good proteins (fish, poultry, beans), just enough good, low-glycemic carbohydrates to meet your energy expenditure (whole grains, vegetables, fruits), and plenty of good fats (avocados, nuts, seeds, olive oil, fish oil, flax oil).
- Stop the intake of alcohol, sugar, refined carbohydrates, fat-free foods, processed food, preservatives, additives, fast foods, junk foods, soft drinks,[46] and artificial sweeteners.
- Stop eating sugar. Studies have found that rats that were addicted to cocaine would choose sugar over cocaine when given the choice.[47] Steer totally clear of sugar. Just as an alcoholic can't have just one drink, a person who is addicted to sugar cannot eat it on occasion without suffering the possibility of a relapse into eating it again on a regular basis. So just stop eating anything with sugar in it. If a sweet taste is needed, use limited portions of fruit.
- Balance your hormones. Read on to learn how.

Part II: Balance Hormones: Lose Fat

7. Most Overweight People Have Hormone Imbalances!

MOST WEIGHT-LOSS CENTERS can't insure long-term success, because they don't look at hormones. Hormones are not usually considered in weight loss programs, but they are critical for success in the long-term. Returning again and again to the weight-loss center makes money for their business, but just makes it harder and harder for you to lose weight if poor metabolism is not corrected. When your hormones are unbalanced, you won't be successful in losing weight over the long haul until you address your hormonal issues.

Weight gain may be the cause of hormone dysfunction. Hormone dysfunction may, in turn, cause weight gain. It's a vicious circle. As you gain that fat, especially belly fat, the fat causes your hormones to become imbalanced. As your hormones become unbalanced, your metabolism gets sick, and you get fatter. The only way out is to correct your hormones.

Most overweight people have hormone imbalances. They will not be able to lose unwanted fat until their hormones have been adjusted. They often have:

1. **Too much insulin.**
2. **Too much estrogen in relation to other hormones.**
3. **An underactive thyroid.**

Next we will examine ach of these imbalances and you will learn strategies for correcting them. See <u>Secrets About Bioidentical Hormones</u>[48] for an in-depth discussion. It can guide you and your physician in how to evaluate hormonal dysfunction.

The first step in the correction of all hormone imbalances is to correct our digestion. Proper digestion is critical to allow proper absorption of the nutrients needed to achieve hormonal balance.

8. Improve Digestion for Hormone Health

GOOD HEALTH BEGINS IN THE GUT. Check for yeast, parasites, intestinal infections, overgrowth of bad bacteria, and other intestinal imbalances and eliminate them. Carbohydrate cravings may be caused by yeast overgrowth in the gut. Intestinal parasites and other intestinal problems may be the reason for gut inflammation.

See a wholistic practitioner who can get your stool tests sent to a reputable lab (like Diagnos-Techs, Metametrix, or Genova), that specializes in finding hard-to-find organisms, so that you can find out what is going on and correct any infections or imbalances. You will need to see a physician who is well-versed in detoxification and anti-aging in order to have these tests performed properly in order to discover any intestinal imbalances. Don't trust stool tests done in a hospital or traditional labs. Unfortunately, parasites hide high in the intestines and can only be found when the intestinal tract is completely emptied. This may require drinking a laxative and then getting a liquid stool sample many hours later, after many bowel movements have occurred. If a problem is found, find out how to eliminate it. After eliminating digestive dysbiosis caused by an overgrowth of yeast, parasites, and bad bacteria, you may still have trouble digesting certain types of food. Then you can look at other reasons for poor digestion—deficient hydrochloric acid, pancreatic enzymes, gall bladder, etc.

Food allergies must be considered. You can get tested for food allergies at specialty labs (Diagnos-Techs, Metametrix, or Genova). It is important to eliminate allergenic foods from your diet. If you eat the same kind of protein a lot, you will be more likely to become allergic to it. Then you will need to eliminate that particular protein to avoid digestive problems. You may be able to come back to it after some time, but maybe not. So it is important to rotate your proteins with each meal and change them each day. If you are having trouble with protein, you can get an amino acid profile that will tell you how you are digesting protein. If you are found to be deficient in certain amino acids, you can tailor your diet to specifically add those amino acids that you are missing by eating specific types of meats or plant proteins.

9. Too Much Insulin

AFTER IMPROVING DIGESTION, THE NEXT STEP in your weight-loss plan is to correct the hormonal imbalances. Let's look first at the common problem of too much insulin.

A. Metabolic syndrome is a major cause and result of obesity. It is the combination of insulin resistance (which increases blood sugar and insulin levels), hypertension, central obesity, and abnormal fats in the blood. It is an inflammatory and toxic process.

The primary component of metabolic syndrome is insulin resistance. It is the result of eating too many carbs, especially processed carbs, with not enough protein and good fats. After you keep eating this way for some time, you develop insulin resistance.

One of the primary reasons for the development of insulin resistance and metabolic syndrome is the consumption of soda pop. Studies have shown that both men and women who drank one diet soda daily had a 36% higher incidence of metabolic syndrome.[49] Sugary beverages play a large factor in the rising tide of metabolic syndrome.[50] High fructose corn syrup is the primary sweetener in soft drinks now. Its use has risen astronomically in the past 30 years. Stanhope reviewed the literature and concluded that, "consumption of fructose has been shown to increase visceral adipose deposition and de novo lipogenesis (DNL), produce dyslipidemia, and decrease insulin sensitivity in older, overweight/obese subjects."[51]

Toxicity is also responsible for causing metabolic syndrome. Toxicity can damage insulin receptors and produce insulin resistance.[52]

Metabolic syndrome affects many of us. It is estimated that 22% of the U.S. adult population or 47 million adults have metabolic syndrome. Up to two-thirds of all women in the menopausal age group have syndrome X (another name for metabolic syndrome). It is more common in African Americans and Hispanics.[53] Menopause and syndrome

X work together to cause age-related disease and disability. Conventional hormone replacement therapy (HRT) (Premarin with or without Provera) will make problems worse.

If your fasting insulin is greater than 10, you may be getting insulin-resistant. Metabolic syndrome eventually worsens into pre-diabetes (fasting blood sugar greater than 99), and then into type 2 diabetes (fasting blood sugar greater than 126).

If your fasting blood sugar is greater than 90, you are heading for metabolic syndrome if you don't correct your lifestyle (eating, sleeping, stress, exercise habits). Don't wait until your fasting blood sugar runs up to 99 to change your ways.

High insulin levels are associated with increased inflammation,[54] blood clotting, abnormal cellular growth, and further insulin resistance. If you are eating normal amounts of food but are tired in the afternoon and getting fatter, you may be hypothyroid or eating too many carbohydrates and developing insulin resistance and reactive hypoglycemia.

The bigger your belly, the worse your metabolic syndrome.[55] The most consistent marker for metabolic syndrome is a waist size greater than 40 inches in men and greater than 35 inches in women. Belly fat produces inflammation. Inflammation interferes with normal insulin action in fat and muscle cells. This is why people with a lot of belly fat have more insulin resistance and why insulin resistance is associated with belly fat.[56] Belly fat and a high ratio of fat to muscle set the stage for insulin resistance, which leads to high insulin levels. Insulin resistance is a major cause of obesity. It also increases risk of cancer[57] and heart disease.[58] It can be improved through lifestyle changes.

B. This is what happens when you have insulin resistance. The muscle cells have difficulty taking in sugar, blood sugar increases, and the fat cells take in the excess sugar and store it as fat. The result is that you get fat and tired. If you don't stop this process, it will lead to a variety of health problems.

When you repeatedly eat a lot of high-glycemic foods, blood sugars go very high, and the muscle cells, red blood cells, and all the other cells in the body become totally saturated with sugar (glycinated). Then the insulin receptors (doors on the cells where sugar can enter) on the muscle cells and other cells begin to malfunction. If excess sugar continues to be eaten, the muscle cells may reduce the number of insulin receptors to try to keep the excess sugar out, thus becoming more resistant to insulin. When the sugar can't get into the muscle cells because the insulin receptors (doors) have malfunctioned and decreased in number, sugar in the bloodstream rises. This causes the pancreas to secrete more insulin in an attempt to get enough sugar into the muscle cells. Then you have a vicious circle, where increased insulin causes increased sugar saturation, which produces increased receptor resistance.

The fat cells store the sugar as fat. This fat will remain in the fat cells as long as the muscle cells remain resistant to insulin. Unlike the muscle cells, the fat cells of insulin-resistant people are all too happy to take in that sugar and store it. When insulin can't store sugar in the muscle cells, it will store any excess sugar in the liver or fat cells. It is a mechanism that evolved to store fat that could be used for energy in times of famine. You get fat, because the fat cells are getting bigger as they store the sugar as fat. But you feel tired, because the muscle cells can't take in the sugar, even when they need it. When the blood becomes saturated with insulin, the insulin-resistant body will not release significant fat stores, even when a person restricts their calorie intake and exercises.

C. Insulin resistance leads to diabetes, cancer, heart disease.

High insulin wrecks your metabolism. When insulin levels rise to higher than normal levels, and insulin resistance occurs, damage occurs to the metabolism. This disrupts the other hormones and biochemical reactions in the cells.

If you have insulin resistance you may develop diabetes if you don't change your ways quickly. When your muscle cells have closed and reduced their number of doors (insulin receptors), you have developed insulin resistance. Insulin resistance may progress into type 2 diabetes, where the pancreas is secreting more and more insulin. At this point, the disease may be reversible. But eventually, if you don't correct faulty eating patterns, your pancreas will totally burn out from overproducing insulin. Then it can't produce enough insulin to live. Then you have type 1 diabetes and require insulin injections. At this point the disease is irreversible and fatal. You develop vascular disease. You go blind. You lose your kidneys. You lose circulation to the extremities, heart, and brain.

High insulin levels increase cancer risk because insulin is an incredibly powerful growth stimulant. (High insulin levels accelerate cell growth and division.) It is important to keep insulin levels low to keep insulin receptors sensitive and to avoid weight gain and the development of chronic and degenerative diseases.

High insulin levels also increase risk for development of heart disease because insulin resistance is responsible for high lipid levels and is related to the inflammation that causes arterial plaque buildup.

D. Let's prevent/reduce insulin resistance.

We know that we need to exercise. But exercise isn't as helpful unless we also correct our diet. This requires a change of lifestyle to make these dietary and exercise changes a permanent way of life. Let's teach all of our children to exercise and eat properly, so that we can prevent them from becoming insulin-resistant, sick, and fat. Physical Education should be a part of every school program.

Insulin resistance often starts in childhood. To lower obesity rates, start with the children.[59] [60] Children have a greater chance of normalizing their weight than do overweight adults who have become sedentary and overeat. Children gain weight because of being overfed and not being taken out to exercise at the playground and the pool. If children are eating too many carbohydrates and not enough protein and fat, they will begin to develop insulin resistance, gaining fat, especially belly fat. As children become fat, parents may put them on a diet. Diets usually focus on lowering fat, which makes them eat even more carbohydrates, resulting in even more body fat and under-nourishment. They lose lean muscle and become more insulin-resistant. These diets prepare them to struggle with weight and hormonal imbalance for the rest of their lives.

10. Control Carbohydrates

***LET'S LEARN EXACTLY HOW TO EAT** to prevent or reverse insulin resistance and other hormonal imbalances.* Let's look first at carbohydrates. Then we will examine fats. We will see how dangerous it is to eat low-carb and low-fat diets as far as our hormones are concerned. Then we will learn exactly how to balance protein, fats, and carbs to balance our hormones.

A. Eat the right amount of carbohydrate.

Don't eat more carbohydrates than your body needs to produce energy. Excess carbohydrates lead people on the path to insulin resistance and diabetes. Eat just enough carbs for the energy that you use. If you are sedentary, eat very few. If you are working out two hours a day, then you will need more. The carbs that you don't use are stored as fat.

But don't eliminate carbs completely. Your brain needs glucose. You get glucose primarily from eating carbs. If you go on a starvation diet, your body will take protein from your muscles to make glucose to feed the brain.[61] You don't want to do that. You don't want to lose muscle mass. This decreases your metabolism and makes it harder and harder to lose fat.

B. Eat the right kind of carbs. Paying attention to the

type of carbohydrates eaten is just as important as limiting their quantity. It is better to eat carbohydrates that digest more slowly (low glycemic), so that blood sugar levels remain stable. The speed at which sugars can be broken down into glucose affects the rate at which insulin will rise. The faster the carbohydrates are broken down, the faster insulin will rise.

Glycemic index is a measure of how quickly food becomes sugar in the blood. Lower glycemic-index carbs take longer to break down. Therefore it is best to eat carbohydrates with a lower glycemic index. Foods that are less refined have lower glycemic indexes. The body will be able to use low-glycemic carbohydrates more efficiently to produce energy. Low-

Fat Loss Secrets that Really Work! 31

glycemic foods include whole grains, fruits like apples and berries, vegetables, and legumes. Look for a list of low-glycemic foods.

Stay away from white foods, which are usually high-glycemic. Eating more than a small amount of foods containing white sugar, white flour, white rice, or white potatoes will send blood sugar levels skyrocketing and then plummeting a couple hours later, resulting in fluctuating energy levels and insulin resistance. This is a problem for a person who likes to snack on food from vending machines. If a person is already insulin-resistant, he or she will react even more strongly to high glycemic foods than someone who has not developed insulin resistance. Instead of white and processed foods, eat darker colored foods like butternut squash, yams, brown rice, lentils, beans, and other whole grains and beans.

Glycemic load is the amount of carbohydrate eaten. For instance, you can eat one date, which has a very high glycemic index, without raising your glycemic load much. But as you eat more and more dates, your glycemic load will rise proportionately. If you can't stop yourself from gorging on high-glycemic-index foods like dates, it is better to avoid them completely. Avoid a high glycemic load by eating smaller amounts of carbohydrates and eating those with a lower glycemic index. This is the key to avoiding insulin resistance and reversing it if it has already developed.

C. Check your carbohydrate metabolism. You

can get an "Organix Comprehensive Profile" from Metametrix labs[62] that looks at the body's cellular metabolic processes and the efficiency of metabolic function. Dr. Eve Bralley describes the test like this, "The Organix is a simple, non-invasive urine collection that addresses several body systems, allows for the design of specific and individualized therapy, and can help guide you to further testing."[63] To get an even more comprehensive health view including carbohydrate metabolism, Metametrix offers the "Women's Health Profile" complex of tests. It measures organic acids, fatty acids, serum lipid peroxides, markers of metabolic syndrome, and estrogen. It can also help assess risk factors associated with genetics, biochemical imbalances, and environmental influences. These tests will show you where you are blocked from being able to digest carbohydrates. They will tell you the enzyme that is deficient and what you need to do to correct it. It might be mercury or some other kind of toxicity that is blocking your carbohydrate metabolism. This is how toxicity makes you fat.

D. Avoid artificial sweeteners. Artificial sweeteners are just as bad as sugar when it comes to raising insulin levels. There are receptors in both the mouth and in the gut that sense any kind of sweet taste. When these receptors sense a sweet taste, they signal the pancreas to secrete insulin.[64] If you must use a sweetener, use a little bit of honey. Honey is anti-glycemic and a whole food.

E. Alcohol harms us in many ways. You can drink grape juice or take Resveratrol to get the benefits of drinking wine without the harmful effects of alcohol. A few ways that it harms us are:

1. Alcohol decreases the production of testosterone in men's testes.[65] [66]
2. Alcohol increases estrogen.[67] People who drink every day can develop estrogen dominance, because the empty calories in alcohol cause belly fat which turns testosterone into estrogen. This is why men who drink a lot have that beer belly and large breasts. They are becoming feminized because they produce less testosterone and the little testosterone that they do have is turned into estrogen.
3. Alcohol increases the risk of breast cancer in women.[68]
4. Alcohol decreases fertility.[69]
5. People who drink more than two drinks a week are more likely to develop atrophy of the brain.[70]
6. Alcohol can cause loss of muscle mass, too.[71]

F. Low-carb diets are harmful over time. If you avoid carbs, you will lower insulin initially. This causes short-term weight loss. But the longer low-carb diets are followed, the more hormonal imbalance occurs. Some problems with low-carb diets include:

1. On low-carb diets less fiber is eaten, increasing estrogen. Fiber is necessary to carry away excess estrogen.[72]
2. People who are on low-carb diets often eat more grilled and smoked meat, which is carcinogenic[73] and increases the incidence of heart disease.[74] Meats with nitrates and nitrites impair hormones.[75]
3. Low-carb diets are usually too high in fat. When you eat a diet that has too many calories from fat (60-70%), Growth Hormone production will be diminished.[76]
4. Low-carb diets are linked to diabetes when followed long-term.[77]

11. Low-Fat Diets Impair Hormones and Health.

NOW THAT WE HAVE SEEN how important it is to eat the right amount and type of carbohydrates in order to prevent insulin resistance, let's turn our attention to fats. Cutting good fats out of your diet can severely damage your health and metabolism. People who eat a low-fat diet reduce protein and essential fats and increase carbs. A low-fat diet leads to the hormone imbalances of insulin resistance, estrogen excess, high cortisol, and thyroid problems. A low-fat diet also lowers testosterone,[78] growth hormone, sex hormones,[79] and DHEA.[80] These hormonal imbalances cause belly fat and inflammation. Inflammation leads to heart disease and many other degenerative diseases.[81] If the diet is not supplying enough proteins and fats, the body will break down its own muscles and bones to use as building blocks to make hormones.

But we can't be healthy by eating just any old fats. We need to learn how to exclude the bad fats and include the good fats in our diets. So what *are* bad fats and what are good fats?

The bad fats include:
- **Hydrogenated fats.**
- **Trans-fats.**
- **Fats in the food at fast-food restaurants.**
- **Fats in processed food.**
- **Fats in restaurant salad dressings.**
- **Margarine.**
- **Vegetable oils high in omega-6 fats.**

These bad fats clog the arteries. They form the small LDL which gets deposited in the arteries. When we eat bad fats, health destruction occurs at the most basic cellular level. Eating bad fats causes insulin resistance and increased risk for diabetes.[82]

Vegetable oils that are too high in Omega-6 fats are highly inflammatory. They block thyroid function by blocking the absorption of iodine in the gut[83] and blocking the conversion of the inactive thyroid hormone, T4 to the active form, T3.[84]

Avoid trans-fats (hydrogenated oils) at all costs.
Trans-fats are not foods. They are chemicals. Trans-fats will be stored in the fat and the body cannot eliminate them. Hydrogenated oils are linked to increased risk for heart disease.[85] They are also linked to lowered testosterone.[86]

The good fats include:
- **Butter.**
- **Olive oil.**
- **Flax oil.**
- **Oils from avocados, nuts, and seeds.**
- **Fish and krill oil.**

The good fats make healthy cell membranes. Health at the cellular level is very important. Do everything you can to help your cells work better. Eating good fats is crucial to cellular health. If the cell membranes aren't working properly, the cells can't take in the good stuff and get rid of the bad stuff. Eat cholesterol-rich foods like shrimp and shellfish (unless farmed). Cholesterol-rich foods should be an important part of your diet if you want to balance your hormones. These fats are needed to form the large LDL part of our cholesterol. This does *not* get deposited in the arteries. LDL flows right through the arteries and doesn't stick.

Without the good fats, our health will decline rapidly. Good fats are essential for the building of hormones and the cell walls of every cell in your body.

We need to eat butter, full-fat dairy, healthy monounsaturated fatty acids (MUFA's) like olive oil, avocados, seeds, and nuts. Essential fatty acids come from these foods. These essential fats allow us to absorb calcium, which is needed to make strong bones. Essential fats are used to make steroid hormones, like estrogen, progesterone, and testosterone.

12. *Balance* Your Diet for Hormone Health

CONTROL YOUR CARB INTAKE AND EAT PLENTY OF PROTEINS, VEGETABLES, AND GOOD FATS.

Eating this way helps you to overcome insulin resistance. Eating this way balances the two hormones that control your blood sugar. These two hormones are insulin and glucagon. Let's see how this works.

Insulin is released in response to carbohydrates. Insulin resistance prevents stored body fat from being released, even when a person undergoes severe calorie restriction, such as crash dieting. If there is more insulin than glucagon, more food will be stored as fat. This is why we want to eat less of foods that increase insulin. That means controlling the proportion of carbs that we eat.

Glucagon is released in response to protein and low blood sugar. Glucagon causes fat loss. Glucagon opens up fat cells so that fat can be burned. If there is relatively more glucagon than insulin, more food will be used as building materials or fuel. This means that we need to eat plenty of protein to balance the carbs that we eat.

Neither excessive insulin nor glucagon is released in response to nonstarchy vegetables and healthy fats. If fats or nonstarchy vegetables are eaten alone, it won't affect either insulin or glucagon. Eating plenty of fats and nonstarchy vegetables is important to give us the building blocks for hormones and the vitamins and minerals necessary for the proper functioning of our bodies.

To balance insulin and glucagon, eat proteins, fats, nonstarchy vegetables, and a moderate amount of low-glycemic carbohydrates together in the same meal. When carbohydrates are eaten without fats, the insulin level goes too high as compared to glucagon, and the food is stored as fat. A rule of thumb is to eat about as much protein as the size of your fist at every meal. Include the good fats, nonstarchy vegetables, and just the right amount of carbohydrate for the energy that you will burn off.

It is impossible to overeat when eating proteins and fat. CCK (Cholecystokinin) is a hormone secreted from the intestinal walls in response to proteins and fats. CCK causes the gallbladder to contract and to secrete bile to absorb fats. CCK goes to the brain and lets it know that the body is being fed. Too much CCK causes nausea. CCK makes it impossible to overeat when you eat proteins and fats. Digestion of carbohydrates does not cause CCK production.

When eating carbohydrates alone, there is no feeling of satiety until the carbohydrates are converted in the liver to glucose which goes to the brain and signals satiety. This takes about twenty minutes and allows you to overeat carbohydrates easily. *Eating the proteins and fats on your plate first will help you to avoid overeating.* This will get that CCK hormone going to your brain.

Specific foods to decrease glucose and insulin:

- **Onions** lower glucose by competing with insulin, increasing insulin activity.
- **Brewer's yeast** is high in chromium which helps insulin bind to the cell receptors.
- **Cinnamon** may act as an insulin substitute and reduces blood sugar 20 to 30 percent.
- **Olive oil** improves blood sugar control while lowering triglycerides.
- **Beans, legumes, and nuts** have fiber which improves glucose tolerance and insulin sensitivity.
- **Mangoes** have a low glycemic index, high fiber, and high enzymes.

Balance proteins, low-glycemic carbs, and good fats. This way of eating balances your insulin levels and heals your metabolism. When you first begin to eat this way, you may actually gain weight for awhile. Do not be discouraged. If you continue on with this healthy way of eating, your metabolism will finally be able to heal. After a period of time, you will notice that you are losing weight and that all of your health problems are improving.

When you get your insulin and glucose levels balanced, you will have more willpower. Your brain won't urge you to eat so often. It will become easier to eat correctly, to exercise, and do things that are good for you that you couldn't do before.

13. Estrogen Dominance

THE SECOND MAJOR HORMONE that becomes unbalanced when we gain weight is estrogen. Overweight people usually have too much estrogen in relation to their other hormones. This is called estrogen dominance.

Excess belly fat in both men and women causes increased estrogen. The belly fat increases estrogen by secreting an enzyme called aromatase. In both men and women, this aromatase, which is secreted by the belly fat, turns their testosterone into estrogen.

In women, this estrogen created by the belly fat increases their risk for breast cancer and endometrial cancer.[87] This estrogen from the belly fat decreases growth hormone,[88] increases oxidative stress,[89] and decreases glutathione production (the most important anti-oxidant).[90]

Too much estrogen in men causes breast enlargement [91] **and prostate inflammation.**[92] Men need some estrogen, but when they have too much in relation to their testosterone and progesterone, they too experience a hormonal imbalance. Whether this happens to women or men, it is called estrogen dominance. Men and women become more estrogen dominant through taking in xenoestrogens (toxins from the environment), production of estrogen from body fat, bad estrogen metabolism, and with the loss of testosterone and progesterone caused by aging. This causes breast enlargement (gynecomastia) in men. Estrogen dominance may also cause prostate inflammation and swelling. As time goes on, estrogen dominance worsens. The intake of toxic chemicals from the environment and altered food supply are huge culprits in the rising tide of estrogen dominance in both sexes.

A. Excess belly fat makes us get even fatter.

Some belly fat is good. It has a feedback mechanism (leptin) that tells the brain when it has had enough food and turns off hunger. But when the belly fat loads up on toxins, the hunger mechanism becomes broken and the hunger is not turned off. Then the fat begins to accumulate in excess.

Belly fat is the worst type of obesity because it increases the risk for heart disease and other diseases.[93] Belly fat is constantly causing inflammation. This inflammation in turn creates more insulin resistance and more belly fat. This is why it is so important to decrease the belly fat.

You can take supplemental hormones to decrease belly fat and other fat gain. [94] [95] [96] Both men and women may lose fat and gain muscle when they bring up low hormone levels by supplementing with DHEA, Testosterone, Thyroid, and Growth Hormone.

B. Fat-soluble toxins are stored in fat, especially belly fat.

Environmental pesticides from food, xenoestrogens from plastics, and other chemical toxicities are stored in fat. Heavy metals are nearly impossible to avoid. Some people have a huge heavy metal burden, unless they have taken steps to chelate the metals out. To study how to remove toxicity from your body go back and read Book One in the Bioidentical Hormone series, Secrets About Bioidentical Hormones.[97]

Toxicity blocks cell receptors, the doors on the cells that let the hormones come in and do their job. Remove toxicity from your body if you want hormones to work. Use far-infrared saunas, bentonite, chelation, colonics, coffee enemas, cleansing juices and foods, supplements, and wheat-grass juice to remove toxicity.

C. Foods to cleanse metabolic wastes:

Eating these foods will help you to cleanse toxicity from your body:
- Beets.
- Garlic.
- Daikon radish.
- Chard.
- Shallots.
- Artichokes.
- Figs.

- Mustard greens.
- Dandelion.
- Collards.
- Turnips.
- Apples.
- Kale.
- Onions.
- Leeks.
- Beet greens.

D. Obese people have high estrogen in relation to the other hormones. It is called estrogen dominance, and it causes a myriad of health problems.[98]

Estrogen dominance is a huge problem, even for men. American men of all ages today have less testosterone than men of the same age did in previous generations.[99] The amount of stress and insulin resistance is increasing radically. This combination of less testosterone, more stress, and insulin resistance is causing more and more belly fat to appear on men. This belly fat is taking what little testosterone men may have to begin with and turning it into estrogen.

The estrogen works against their testosterone. Having low testosterone increases men's risk for dying younger from heart disease.[100]

In women, estrogen becomes unbalanced when there is too much of it in relationship to progesterone. This can happen at any age. The most common pre-menopausal hormone problem in women is estrogen excess and progesterone deficiency. In an estrogen-dominant state, thyroid hormone function is diminished because estrogen increases thyroid-binding globulin, which binds free thyroid hormone. This creates fatigue and weight gain. Allergies may worsen. Blood clots more easily which may set you up for deep venous thrombosis, a stroke, or embolism. Bile thickens and gallbladder problems develop.

Aging causes weight gain, especially in women.

When women hit menopause, all three sex hormones decline--estrogen, progesterone, and testosterone. In menopause, even though estrogen drops, and the woman is estrogen-deficient, she may still have estrogen dominance, as estrogen may be greater proportionately to progesterone.

When a woman enters menopause, her ovaries shut down. This slows the production of the type of estrogen called estradiol (E2). At menopause, many women develop more body fat in order to produce more estrogen to make up for the lost estrogen as the ovaries stop producing estrogen.[101] Then the main estrogen becomes estrone (E1) from the adrenals and body fat. The risk for breast cancer increases.[102] When estrone is the predominant estrogen, it becomes very hard to lose fat. It becomes a vicious cycle of increasing fat and an inability to lose it.

E. Artificial estrogens make us fat.

Premarin, a hormone made from horse's urine, is a common cause of estrogen dominance. Premarin is a popular treatment for menopausal symptoms. When menopausal women take any type of estrogen without progesterone, estrogen becomes unbalanced in relation to progesterone. Estrogen becomes dominant. Premarin is particularly harmful because it is not a human hormone and cannot be metabolized properly by the human body. The metabolites of a foreign, non-human hormone are potently estrogenic and are not easily removed from the body. Even though substantial evidence has accumulated to prove the harm caused by Premarin,[103] it is still being prescribed by doctors and used by millions of women all over the world.

Whenever the body takes in artificial estrogens like Premarin, birth control-pills, and xenoestrogens (from plastics and other environmental toxins),[104] harmful metabolites are formed when the body breaks them down. Because the body cannot readily excrete these harmful metabolites, they are stored in the fat.

When we ingest a foreign substance that acts like our own hormones, it acts as a "gender bender." This term came from the fact that animals and fish become feminized when they are exposed to these toxins. When we are exposed to gender benders from eating pesticides from non-organic food, we develop estrogen dominance. Dioxin (Agent Orange) is another gender-bender that creates the bad estrogen metabolism that causes cancer.[105] Many people have faulty estrogen metabolism because of the toxicity of gender benders. It is important to check estrogen metabolism[106] and to correct faulty estrogen metabolism. Faulty estrogen metabolism leads to the development of cancer.

Estrogen metabolism can be improved by eating cruciferous vegetables, limiting alcohol intake, and avoiding gender benders.[107] These xenoestrogens are all around us. They all create abnormal estrogen metabolism. They create estrogen dominance which leads to weight gain and increased risk for cancer. They cause girls to enter puberty earlier than those of previous generations.[108] Avoid the intake of gender benders by avoiding pollution of all kinds. Avoid drinking out of plastic bottles. Eat organic food. Filter your water. Move away from high-voltage power lines and polluted air. Move as far away from cities and cell-phone towers as you possibly can.

F. Symptoms of estrogen dominance:

- Irritability/mood swings/anxiety, PMS.
- Salt and fluid retention.
- Blood clotting.
- Allergic reaction.
- Increased production of body fat.
- Food cravings.
- Hot flashes.
- Irregular periods.
- Depression.
- Water retention/bloating.
- Sleep disturbance.
- Headaches.
- Fatigue.
- Short term memory loss.
- Craving for sweets.
- Uterine fibroids.
- Breast pain, breast swelling (all month long), fibrocystic breasts.
- Breast, uterine, ovarian cancer.

- Endometriosis, polycystic ovaries.
- Increased cholesterol and triglyceride levels.
- Interference with thyroid hormone function (weight gain and exhaustion).

G. How to treat estrogen dominance.

- Optimize hormones, especially sex hormones.
- Reduce toxicity—decrease xenoestrogens with zeolite, Calcium D-Glucarate.
- Reduce stress and causes for adrenal dysfunction.
- Exercise regularly.
- Change unhealthy dietary habits and decrease insulin resistance.
- Take fiber with the highest-fat meal of the day to eliminate excess estrogen and toxicity.
- Add two to four grams of fish oil per day to lower inflammation.
- Treat abnormal estrogen metabolism with DIM and calcium D-Glucarate.

For estrogen dominance in women, the treatment is bioidentical progesterone. Progesterone counterbalances the effects of estrogen. Too much estrogen and too little progesterone (estrogen dominance) may cause women to become too nervous because it drops GABA levels in the brain. GABA is a neurotransmitter that keeps us calm and helps us to sleep.

Estrogen dominance worsens as women age. It may begin in the twenties, especially with the use of synthetic hormones used for birth control. Unopposed estrogen causes PMS, growth of uterine fibroids, endometrial cancer, and fibrocystic disease of the breast. If the problem of progesterone insufficiency is not addressed, estrogen dominance can get out of control.

We can balance our hormones safely by using bioidentical hormones. These are supplemental hormones that exactly match the hormones that are made by our bodies. Because they are identical to those made by our bodies, bioidentical hormones may be used safely. Attention must be paid to optimizing estrogen metabolism. They should be used in the proper amounts to correct imbalances and in the proper timing to mimic the hormonal status of young, healthy people.

For more information on how to use bioidentical hormones, read the other books in the "Bioidentical Hormone" series.[109] [110] [111]

It is important to find a physician who really understands women's hormones, knows when and how to check hormone levels, and is not afraid to prescribe BHRT. Many physicians will simply ignore women's complaints that are caused by estrogen dominance and chalk it up to emotions.

Other physicians may check estrogen, FSH, and LH levels. But progesterone levels may not be checked. As estrogen levels fluctuate quite a bit, if estrogen is low on the day it is measured, the physician may prescribe estrogen. This will make everything worse when estrogen is dominant in relation to progesterone. The major part of estrogen dominance may be from the xenoestrogen load which is impossible to measure and/or from estrogen metabolites.

A physician may erroneously diagnose low estrogen when using a blood test for a woman who is using a transdermal cream. He/she may then prescribe increased estradiol even though the woman is actually estrogen-dominant. This is because the wrong test has been used. To measure estrogen in tissues, the most accurate test is saliva.

Another problem may be that the physician ignores the ratio of estrogen to progesterone. Most post-menopausal women are estrogen-deficient and estrogen-dominant (in relation to progesterone) at the same time. Absolute levels of estrogen and progesterone are not as important as keeping the two hormones balanced.

Balancing the two hormones is critical to maintaining health. Too *much* progesterone can also be a problem, so avoid taking too much progesterone. Keep the two hormones balanced to prevent insulin resistance.[112]

Lifestyle changes may be enough to correct the problem in men, as testosterone levels will rise when insulin levels and body fat drop. If testosterone levels are still low after improving weight and lifestyle, begin treating the low-testosterone state with hCG or testosterone. If estrogen levels are still increased after diet and lifestyle changes, use an aromatase inhibitor (anastrozole). If 16-hydroxy metabolites are increased, use DIM.[113]

For men, estrogen excess can be overcome by using aromatase inhibitors like Arimidex, which control estrogen. The best diet to eat to optimize testosterone is to eat plenty of good fat. 40% of the calories in the diet should come from fat in order to have the building blocks to make plenty of testosterone. A low-fat diet is particularly destructive to adequate testosterone (and all other hormone) production.

Calcium D-Glucarate corrects estrogen excess caused by synthetic hormones.[114] Because of all the synthetic hormones and xenoestrogens coming in from environmental pollutants like plastic, cosmetics, insecticides, and pesticides, most people have a huge toxic load of chemical hormones circulating in the body, and there's no way for the body to get rid of them.

Calcium D-Glucarate helps the body to eliminate a lot of these synthetic hormones, carcinogens, and tumor-promoters. Women who are trying to get pregnant may get pregnant after using Calcium D-Glucarate for a few months. It helps to decrease excess estrogen quickly. Make sure to use enough. Be careful though, as it may interfere with some prescription antidepressants. Zeolite also corrects estrogen dominance caused by xenoestrogens. You can find these products on the internet.

We have covered the first two major hormonal imbalances that are responsible for weight gain, insulin and estrogen. Having an underactive thyroid is the third major hormonal imbalance that must be addressed if we want to normalize weight. But before correcting the thyroid, we must have healthy adrenals. Let's find out next how to normalize our adrenal functioning.

14. Heal the Adrenals, Then the Thyroid

BEFORE TREATING THE THYROID, first address adrenal fatigue or exhaustion. Often thyroid disorders appear seemingly out of the blue right after a stressful event like a divorce or losing one's job. There is a reason for this. Stress causes the adrenals to secrete more hormones. When the stress is chronic and unrelenting, eventually the adrenals burn out. When the adrenals are dysfunctional, thyroid hormone can't work right either.

There are some symptoms that may help you to distinguish between thyroid and adrenal dysfunction. If you wake up tired in the morning, are tired all day long, and have poor, restless sleep at night, you probably have adrenal dysfunction. You feel wired but tired. You may fall asleep in the middle of the day, even while driving. You may crave salt. Conversely, if you *only* get tired in the afternoon, have dry skin, are constipated, and sleep poorly, you probably have thyroid dysfunction.

If you ramp up the metabolism with thyroid medication and the adrenals aren't functioning well, you will get poor results. By improving adrenal functioning first, thyroid treatment will be more effective.

So before treating the thyroid, let's address the adrenals and look at the role of stress. Oftentimes, reducing stress and healing the adrenals will allow thyroid function to improve adequately, without any other intervention.

Let's see what happens to the glands that secrete hormones to deal with stress—the adrenals. Let's look at two major hormones that are produced by the adrenals—cortisol and DHEA. Let's examine how stress affects our hormones.

A. Cortisol is a stress hormone produced by the adrenals. It is a most important hormone in the body because it keeps us alive. Without it, we would die from any stress. When we get sick, cortisol increases to stimulate the immune system to

46 Fat Loss Secrets that Really Work!

fight the illness. Cortisol tells the body to fight off any kind off threat. When it becomes chronically low, the immune system can't work and we may fall prey to chronic deficiency of the immune system and get diseases like infections and cancer.

Chronic stress produces adrenal dysfunction. Impaired levels of cortisol (from adrenal burn-out) may lead to weight gain and other health issues. This in turn causes imbalances in all of the other hormones.

Gaining weight, stress, and aging make cortisol rise initially. This high cortisol encourages the development of osteoporosis, insulin resistance, high cholesterol, insomnia, and depression. High cortisol levels cause cravings for coffee, sugar, sweets, soft drinks, and salty snacks.

If cortisol has been high enough for long enough, the adrenals will give out and you will go into adrenal fatigue and exhaustion, disorders that are not recognized at all by traditional doctors. Most of us have adrenal dysfunction because we all are under so much stress. As time goes on, the adrenals can no longer produce enough cortisol to deal with the demands of life. You become more and more tired, especially so in the morning. It becomes difficult to even get out of bed. Drinking coffee and taking stimulants is counter-productive, as this stresses the adrenals even more.

Eventually you may totally collapse if you don't change your lifestyle and lower your stress.[115] Other ways to heal the adrenals include vitamins (particularly vitamin C), herbs, and small physiological doses of natural cortisol for three to six months or so. Treatment methods are discussed in detail in my book, Secrets About Bioidentical Hormones![116]

Adrenal health is very important to the healthy functioning of all of the other endocrine organs. When we are under chronic stress, the building blocks that would normally be used to make all of the other hormones are used instead to form cortisol. This is called cortisol steal.[117] The results are impaired insulin sensitivity, impaired thyroid (reduced conversion of T4 to T3), decreased sex hormones, immune suppression, high blood sugar, high blood pressure, high lipids, bone loss, and belly fat.

In stage 3-4 adrenal dysfunction, the production of sex hormones is significantly impaired. Estrogen, progesterone, and testosterone production all will be affected. In cycling women, this may cause irregular periods. In both men and women their sexual desire will diminish.

B. Progesterone drops with stress. Pre-menopausal women under stress have difficulty forming enough progesterone, and they become more and more estrogen-dominant. The most common cause for the symptoms of PMS is luteal insufficiency. In luteal insufficiency, the egg sac does not produce adequate progesterone.

Many women in their 30's and early 40's who are under chronic stress become perimenopausal. The stress produces anovulatory cycles. Because the stress is blocking ovulation, they have no egg sac and are extremely progesterone-deficient.

It is very important to keep women's progesterone levels high enough throughout the second half of the menstrual cycle. It is anti-inflammatory. If we are depleting progesterone through increased stress, inflammation increases all throughout the body, which leads to many health problems. Progesterone balances estrogen, improves immunity, prevents negative effects of estrogen (especially on the uterine lining and breast), and protects your brain and nervous system.

C. Stress drops men's testosterone. Increased stress causes increased belly fat, which decreases men's already-too-low testosterone, while increasing estrogen as well. This belly fat causes inflammation as well, which increases incidence of heart problems and many other diseases.

Young men in their 20's and 30's often have very low testosterone levels when they are under a lot of stress. These men may benefit from an improved diet, decreased stress, and increased zinc. There are natural substances that may raise testosterone without lowering sperm count, if they want to reproduce. HCG will increase testosterone levels and support increased spermatogenesis. Testosterone therapy may be used if they do not care about keeping their sperm count up. It may be used temporarily until they can build their own production back up by improving lifestyle.

D. To balance your hormones, control stress. This will help to normalize cortisol levels and heal adrenals. If stress remains high, the brain will be damaged. The hippocampus, which supervises the master controller, the hypothalamus, degenerates from chronic stress and increased cortisol. In chronic stress, adrenalin is also elevated, and the sympathetic nervous system dominates the parasympathetic nervous system. This sympathetic nervous system domination produces type-A behavior and time-urgency, which shorten life. Phosphatidylserine may help this problem because it lowers high cortisols that are common in people with high stress levels. It is especially helpful at night to treat the sleep disorder caused by high cortisol.

Stress is multi-faceted. Stress isn't just disharmony at home, although that is the worst stress. To remove stress you need to eliminate anything that creates fear, worry, anxiety, depression, pain syndromes, eating food to which you have allergies or gluten intolerance, toxic exposure, heavy metals, inflammation, low blood sugar, electromagnetic fields, nutritional deficiencies, and inadequate or disturbed sleep. You have to look at anything that raises cortisol levels.

Learn to control your reaction to stress and remove stress from your life. Meditate. Reframe your reaction to stresses. Do whatever it takes. Just reduce the stress.

Get to bed early and sleep as much as possible. Sleep is critical. Without adequate sleep, you have decreased melatonin and Growth Hormone. You will gain weight, and show an increased stress profile with high levels of cortisol and a decline in DHEA. This

increases cardiovascular risk, insulin resistance, adrenal problems, and disrupts the thyroid.

E. DHEA declines with stress, aging, and weight gain.
DHEA is another adrenal hormone that can be negatively affected by chronic stress. If your DHEA is low, it may indicate that you are heading for adrenal fatigue and exhaustion which can be diagnosed by measuring cortisol levels throughout the day.

DHEA balances cortisol. Cortisol is catabolic—tissues break down. DHEA is anabolic—tissues build. DHEA is necessary to balance cortisol. It restores everything that cortisol has used up to deal with the stress. When your cortisol is chronically high and you don't have enough DHEA, you will burn out your adrenals because you aren't restoring the adrenals.

Low DHEA levels increase your desire to binge on carbs. It affects serotonin, which affects appetite. When DHEA is low, serotonin levels drop and carbohydrate cravings increase.

Supplementing with DHEA when levels are low is helpful in reversing insulin resistance.[118] By supplementing with DHEA, it makes it easier to control our weight.

Make sure you are taking a supplement that provides sulphur, such as MSM, because sulfur is necessary to store DHEA. B-vitamins, like choline and inositol, are also important. Inositol helps with anxiety and insomnia. Choline helps to detox the liver and improves the functioning of the gall bladder.

When you have enough DHEA, you are more likely to have a sense of well-being, less depression, and better sex drive. Women need to be careful not to take too much DHEA, as too much can cause masculinization, like facial hair. Women can start at 5 mg per day and work up to 25 mg a day. Men can take up to 50 mg a day.

15. An Underactive Thyroid

Now LET'S LOOK AT THE THIRD MAJOR HORMONAL IMBALANCE responsible for weight gain, having too little active thyroid hormone. After stabilizing and supporting the adrenals, the thyroid can be addressed. Thyroid affects the other hormones and the other hormones affect the thyroid. As your thyroid problems worsen, so do all of your other hormonal imbalances. Insulin resistance worsens. Inflammation increases. Stress on your adrenals increases. As all of these other hormones worsen because of the thyroid problem, the thyroid problem gets worse. This causes incidence of all degenerative diseases to increase.

It is very important to correct the thyroid problem if you want to lose weight and improve your health. Your metabolism may be reduced by as much as 40% when your thyroid isn't working optimally. You can't take up the food to use it for energy. Thyroid hormone is necessary for the cells to utilize oxygen and for the mitochondria (the powerhouses) of the cells to make energy. If your thyroid is working suboptimally, you are more likely to have insulin resistance. Your muscle cells won't be able to take in the glucose (sugar) and use it for energy. Instead it is stored in the fat cells, which makes you fatter. Hypothyroidism increases 16 hydroxy-estrone, which is the more pro-carcinogenic estrogen metabolite and greatly contributes to estrogen dominance. Low thyroid increases the risk for breast cancer in this way. Hypothyroidism produces immune impairment, which increases the risk for all cancers. Low thyroid also increases estrogen because there is less sex-hormone binding globulin. Again this causes estrogen dominance, which may aggravate endometrial cancer or breast cancer.

Common symptoms of hypothyroidism include:

- Low body temperature
- Cold hands and feet
- Constipation
- Puffy eyelids
- Hair loss
- Dry skin

There are many things that you can do to improve your thyroid functioning. Let's look at each of these strategies.

A. Don't eat a low carb diet. Low-carb diets disrupt
thyroid hormone.[119] Researchers found that, "During the low carbohydrate diet rT3 increased and T3 decreased but they remained unchanged during the carbohydrate-rich diet." We will see in a minute how rT3 (reverse T3) blocks thyroid function and the importance of keeping the active thyroid hormone, T3, levels high for optimum functioning.[120]

B. Take the right amount of iodine. You need
enough, but not too much. WTS Med puts out a very good product for the thyroid called Thyroid Px. You can get it through your health-care provider. "Atomidine" is another great source of iodine. It was recommended by Edgar Cayce. Iodine deficiency is a big problem. You can get tested for it. You can also check for bromine. Bromine blocks iodine from forming thyroid hormones. Many people are bromine toxic, especially since most bread manufacturers stopped using iodine and started using bromine. Iodine is good. Bromine is bad because it contributes to halogen toxicity. Sea salt helps to detoxify bromine.

C. Get an accurate diagnosis and treatment.
You can get much worse if you don't receive the right treatment. You need to make sure that your adrenals are functioning well also. You cannot optimize your thyroid without correcting adrenals.[121] Thyroid dysfunction is commonly misdiagnosed or mistreated. The majority of physicians diagnose low thyroid by getting a blood test that measures TSH, or thyroid-stimulating hormone, that is secreted by the pituitary gland in the brain. When this number goes high enough, they will declare you to be hypothyroid. These physicians will often prescribe a medication that contains only T4, the inactive form of thyroid. There are two major problems here.

(1) Many people are sub-clinically hypothyroid. That
means that the thyroid gland is not working optimally, but your TSH hasn't gone up enough to be declared hypothyroid by your doctor. So you just have to wait until the problem gets bad enough and then you can get help. Wouldn't it be better to treat the problem *before* it gets really bad?

(2) The medicine (T4) that your doctor prescribes may not help you, or you may worsen even though blood tests show that you are better.

This problem may arise if you are prescribed T4 (synthroid) and you can't convert it to the T3 that your body can use. Your TSH levels may drop to normal, because your pituitary senses that you have enough T4. The pituitary slows down its stimulation of the thyroid to make T4. *But if you can't convert it to the T3 that the body can use, the T4 that you are taking is useless. You still feel tired and continue to pack on the pounds. If you convert the T4 to false T3 (Reverse T3), you will get even more hypothyroid, even if the blood tests are normal.*

A doctor who really understands the thyroid would not prescribe T4 without first checking blood levels of bioavailable free T3 to find out if you are converting T4 to T3 or not. If you are not able to convert T4 to T3, you need to supplement with T3 in order for thyroid hormone to work in your body.[122] Decreasing the stress on the adrenals may help you to make the conversion of T4 to T3 because increased cortisol blocks the conversion.[123] [124] You may be able to overcome this T4 to T3 conversion problem by using the Wilson's protocol. If your body temperature is consistently low, this protocol may help you.[125]

As women age, they may have more trouble converting T4 to T3. To make the conversion from T4 to T3, an enzyme is needed. The enzymes of perimenopausal women don't work as well. This gets worse when they hit menopause. Subclinical hypothyroidism is quite common after menopause.[126] Nutrients which are important to be able to convert T4 to T3 include iodine, selenium, potassium, iron, zinc, Vitamins A, E, and riboflavin. Adding these nutrients may increase the conversion and make your neurotransmitters in your brain work better, thus decreasing depression. You need enough cortisol, but not too much. You need the right balance of estrogen, progesterone, and testosterone.

If you can't convert T4 to T3 and you take T4, you can make your thyroid problem worse. The T4 that you are taking may be converted to Reverse T3. Reverse T3 causes your metabolism to drop even further and cause you to gain weight. Reverse T3 is bio-inactive. It is the storage form of T3. It looks like T3, only it is exactly backward. It will bind onto the thyroid receptors on the cells, so that T3 can't get into the cells. It takes the place of T3. It doesn't do anything. Stress, selenium deficiency, or Vitamin A deficiency increase the production of Reverse T3. The bottom line here is that if your physician has prescribed T4 only on the basis of the results of a TSH test, without checking Free T4, Free T3, Reverse T3, and antibodies, ask for these tests or find a physician who understands how these thyroid hormones work and will order the tests for you.

D. If you have a lot of Reverse T3, *add selenium, Vitamin A, and decrease stress.* This may
decrease the production of Reverse T3, so that the active T3 can come into the cells and do its job. If you only check T4 and T3 and find that these levels are high, but you still have hypothyroid symptoms, it would be wise to check Reverse T3. If you check Reverse T3, and it is high, T3 is being blocked from being able to go into the cells by the Reverse T3. This Reverse T3 doesn't make energy. It blocks the cell receptors (doors) from being able to take in T3. The definitive treatment is the Wilson's Temperature Syndrome protocol.

E. Get a physical to check your thyroid. You
may have a goiter that has not been diagnosed. There may be a cancer.

F. If you have anti-thyroid antibodies, be sure to try a gluten-free diet. You may have
Hashimoto's thyroiditis. Your physician would have to order an antibodies test to check this out. There is a cross reactivity between gluten antibodies (gliadin) and thyroid antibodies. Look for other reasons for the positive antibodies. It might be because of heavy metals, food allergies, or a neurotransmitter imbalance.

G. Low thyroid is associated with impaired digestion. This causes impaired Phase One digestion. Inadequate
digestion in the stomach causes putrification in the small intestines. You can help this situation with betaine hydrochloride, pepsin, and probiotics. Add one hydrochloric acid capsule 15 minutes before eating. If there is no burning, at the next meal you can add another capsule. Increase until you feel burning, then back down to the last dose. See if chronic heartburn decreases and digestion improves, especially gas.

Part III: Flying into Action

16. Find a Physician Who Will Treat All Hormone Imbalances

***THE CURRENT STANDARD OF CARE** (for most primary-care physicians, endocrinologists, internists, etc.) is to diagnose and treat only extreme hormonal imbalances.* Anti-aging physicians and alternative medical physicians treat mild, moderate, and severe hormonal dysfunctions preventing the deterioration to extreme hormonal imbalances. If you are unable to find a doctor in your area who is willing to treat you with bioidentical hormones for your hormonal deficiencies and imbalances, *be they mild, moderate, or severe,* find a doctor associated with the American Academy of Anti-Aging Medicine (A4M)[127] or American College for Advancement in Medicine (ACAM).[128] These anti-aging and functional medicine doctors are practicing state-of-the-art medicine, the medicine conservative physicians will be practicing in forty years. These doctors will be able to order the tests that you need.

American Academy of Anti-Aging Medicine (A4M)
888-997-0112   http://www.worldhealth.net/

American College for Advancement in Medicine (ACAM)
800-532-3688   http://www.acamnet.org

Look for a caring doctor with a warm heart. Avoid doctors whose only concern is to maximize profits for their HMO. Sidestep also the greedy ones, who maximize profits for themselves. Beware of any who feel that they are superior to you, "the patient," or those who are simply lazy or incompetent. Your goal is to find a physician whose motivation comes from the heart, works hard to be of service to you, who will approach you as a unique person, and will travel with you on your quest for health.

17. Treatment Plan to Balance Hormones

- *START WITH THE GUT.* Eliminate yeast, parasites, and dysbiosis. Avoid eating foods to which you are allergic. Take hydrochloric acid, digestive enzymes, and probiotics as needed. If there are any issues with gluten, adopt a gluten-free diet.
- *Get plenty of sleep.* Get to bed early and sleep as much as possible. Adopt good sleep hygiene.
- *Don't overeat.* Reduce calories by 500 each day to lose 1-2 pounds a week. Take calorie restriction mimetics for more benefits. Eat a nutrient-dense, low-calorie diet.
- *Don't crash diet* (less than 800 calories a day). Yo-yo dieting causes hormonal imbalance.
- *Eat a good breakfast.*
- *Diet and exercise are key.*
- *Balance your diet* with plenty of good proteins (fish, poultry, beans), enough good low-glycemic carbohydrates to meet your energy expenditure (whole grains, vegetables, fruits), and lots of good fats (avocados, nuts, seeds, olive oil, fish oil, flax oil, butter).
- *Don't eat processed foods.* Eat natural, whole foods.
- *Reverse insulin resistance.* Use an exercise program that includes strength training, cardio, and abdominal exercises. Stretch. Don't overtrain. Follow the treatment plan presented in Secrets About Bioidentical Hormones! [129]
- *Use weight loss surgery cautiously* and only for clinically severe and morbid obesity.
- *Some pharmaceuticals, such as Metformin, are important.* Follow your doctor's advice. Supplements may be helpful, but aren't a magic bullet. Many have toxic side effects.
- *Avoid alcohol and all other toxins* like preservatives, pesticides, herbicides, and other xenoestrogens.
- *Treat estrogen dominance in women* with lifestyle changes and bioidentical progesterone *prescribed by a physician.*

- ***Treat estrogen dominance in men*** by raising testosterone levels, decreasing aromatization of testosterone into estrogen, and using DIM to improve estrogen metabolism (bad or ugly hydroxylation).[130] Use lifestyle change, herbs, and supplemental pharmaceuticals as needed.

- ***Address the adrenals before treating the thyroid.***

- ***Reduce stress and cortisol demand*** with yoga, tai chi, meditation, and setting boundaries.

- ***Remove other sources of physical stress*** not often considered, like heavy metals, dental disease, toxicity, etc.

- ***Supplement with DHEA*** if it is low.

- ***Use EPA and DHA*** supplements.

- ***Correct the thyroid*** by seeing a physician who understands complex thyroid problems and will order all the tests, not just TSH. Test free T4, free T3, Reverse T3, and antibodies. Get a physical exam. Treat the specific thyroid problem that exists, even if it is sub-clinical. Make sure that you have the right building blocks to make thyroid hormone and to convert T4 to T3—iodine, selenium, potassium, iron, zinc, Vitamins A, E, and riboflavin.

- ***Balance the sex hormones***—estrogen, progesterone, and testosterone. Use supplemental bioidentical hormones as needed.

- ***Don't be afraid of any initial weight gain that may occur as you correct your metabolism.*** This is only temporary. If you continue to follow these guidelines, your weight will normalize after six months to a year. Don't be in too much of a rush. Allow your body to heal first, and then the fat will drop off as your metabolism begins to work better.

- ***You will lose the fat and keep it off if you use this information!*** If you set your intention to lose the fat and keep it off, with the help of this book, you will succeed. Refer to the book often and the expanded information in <u>Secrets about Bioidentical Hormones!</u> [131] Good luck following the program!

INDEX

abdominal fat 19
allergies 39
anastrozole.......................................44
antidepressants................................44
antioxidants......................................19
anxiety 41
appetite...19
belly fat 27, 29
BHRT 43
bioidentical 42, 54
bioidentical hormones.......................54
bloating...41
blood sugar 27, 30, 31, 35, 36
body fat 19, 29, 35, 37, 41
bones..33
Calcium D-Glucarate.........................44
cancer..27, 29, 42
carbohydrates .19, 27, 29, 30, 31, 35, 36
carcinogens 44
CCK...35
cholesterol..42
cosmetics 44
cravings......................................19, 41
depression 19. 41
detoxification 25
DHEA 19
diabetes 30
diet..29, 33, 44
dieting...19, 35
diets..29
enzymes..36
estrogen..............39, 40, 41, 42, 43, 44
estrogen dominance 42, 43
exercise...42
fatigue...39, 41
fats 26, 35, 36
fiber...19, 36, 42
fibrocystic...42
fibroids..42
fish oil 42
FSH...43
gallbladder 35, 40
glucagon 35
glucose 36
glycemic index 30
glycemic load....................................31
gynecomastia. 37
headaches 41
heart 29, 54
hot flashes...41

hypertension.....................................26
hypothyroid 27
inflammation..................25, 27, 29, 37
inflammatory 26
insulin ...19, 24, 26, 27, 28, 29, 30, 31, 36, 44
insulin resistance ...19, 26, 27, 28, 29, 31, 35
lead 30
LH 43
liver 19, 28, 36
low-glycemic carbs 30, 36
maintenance......................................19
memory..41
menopause..27
metabolic syndrome 26, 27
metabolism..28
metabolites 40, 43
mood 41
obesity 19, 27
ovaries 42
overweight 24
pain 42
pesticides 44
plaque...29
PMS..41, 42
Premarin.....................................27, 40
progesterone 39, 40, 42, 43
prostate 37
protein....................26, 29, 33, 35, 36
Provera 27
receptors....................................28, 29, 36
serotonin 19
sleep 19, 41
stimulant 19, 29
stress 23, 42
stroke 40
synthetic hormones...........................44
thyroid 24, 39, 42
toxic 26, 44
transdermal 43
tryptophan...19
tumor..44
unopposed estrogen..........................40
urine...43
waist size 27
weight.........................19, 29, 39, 42
weight gain 29, 39, 42
xenoestrogens.............................37, 43
yeast...36

REFERENCES

[1] Ahima RS. Digging deeper into obesity. *J Clin Invest. 2011 Jun 1;121(6):2076-9.*

[2] St Jeor ST, Howard BV, Prewitt TE, Bovee V, Bazzarre T, Eckel RH; Nutrition Committee of the Council on Nutrition, Physical Activity, and Metabolism of the American Heart Association. Dietary protein and weight reduction: a statement for healthcare professionals from the Nutrition Committee of the Council on Nutrition, Physical Activity, and Metabolism of the American Heart Association. *Circulation. 2001 Oct 9;104(15):1869-74.*

[3] Moyad MA. Fad diets and obesity--Part IV: Low-carbohydrate vs. low-fat diets. *Urol Nurs. 2005 Feb;25(1):67-70.*

[4] Dansinger ML, Gleason JA, Griffith JL, Selker HP, Schaefer EJ. Comparison of the Atkins, Ornish, Weight Watchers, and Zone diets for weight loss and heart disease risk reduction: a randomized trial. *JAMA. 2005 Jan 5;293(1):43-53.*

[5] Dietary Reference Intakes for Energy, Carbohydrate, Fiber, Fat, Fatty Acids, Cholesterol, Protein, and Amino Acids. *Institute of Medicine of the National Academies, Food and Nutrition Board. September 5, 2002.*

[6] Colvin RH, Olson SB. A descriptive analysis of men and women who have lost significant weight and are highly successful at maintaining the loss. *Addict Behav. 1983;8(3):287-95.*

[7] Klem ML, Wing RR, McGuire MT, Seagle HM, Hill JO. A descriptive study of individuals successful at long-term maintenance of substantial weight loss. Am J Clin Nutr. 1997 Aug;66(2):239-46.

[8] http://www.nwcr.ws/Research/default.htm

[9] Masuo K, Rakugi H, Ogihara T, Lambert GW. Different mechanisms in weight loss-induced blood pressure reduction between a calorie-restricted diet and exercise. *Hypertens Res. 2011 Aug 4.*

[10] Levitsky DA, Pacanowski CR. Free will and the obesity epidemic. Public *Health Nutr. 2011 Sep 19:1-16.*

[11] Vázquez C, Montagna C, Alcaraz F, Balsa JA, Zamarrón I, Arrieta F, Botella-Carretero JI. Meal replacement with a low-calorie diet formula in weight loss maintenance after weight loss induction with diet alone. *Eur J Clin Nutr. 2009 Oct;63(10):1226-32.*

[12] Chiba T, Tsuchiya T, Komatsu T, Mori R, Hayashi H, Shimokawa I. Development of calorie restriction mimetics as therapeutics for obesity, diabetes, inflammatory and neurodegenerative diseases. *Curr Genomics. 2010 Dec;11(8):562-7.*

[13] Santeusanio F, Di Loreto C, Lucidi P, Murdolo G, De Cicco A, Parlanti N, Piccioni F, De Feo P. Diabetes and exercise. *J Endocrinol Invest. 2003 Sep;26(9):937-40. Review.*

[14] Hopps E, Caimi G. Exercise in obesity management. *J Sports Med Phys Fitness. 2011 Jun;51(2):275-82.*

[15] Seo DI, Jun TW, Park KS, Chang H, So WY, Song W. 12 weeks of combined exercise is better than aerobic exercise for increasing growth hormone in middle-aged women. *Int J Sport Nutr Exerc Metab. 2010 Feb;20(1):21-6.*

[16] Gibala MJ, Little JP, van Essen M, Wilkin GP, Burgomaster KA, Safdar A, Raha S, Tarnopolsky MA. Short-term sprint interval versus traditional endurance training: similar initial adaptations in human skeletal muscle and exercise performance. *J Physiol. 2006 Sep 15;575(Pt 3):901-11.*

[17] de Mello MT, de Piano A, Carnier J, Sanches Pde L, Corrêa FA, Tock L, Ernandes RM, Tufik S, Dâmaso AR. Long-term effects of aerobic plus resistance training on the metabolic syndrome and adiponectinemia in obese adolescents. *J Clin Hypertens (Greenwich). 2011 May;13(5):343-50.*

[18] Walberg JL. Aerobic exercise and resistance weight-training during weight reduction. Implications for obese persons and athletes. *Sports Med. 1989 Jun;7(6):343-56.*

[19] Bodenant M, Kuulasmaa K, Wagner A, Kee F, Palmieri L, Ferrario MM, Montaye M,

Amouyel P, Dallongeville J; for the MORGAM Project. Measures of Abdominal Adiposity and the Risk of Stroke: The Monica Risk, Genetics, Archiving and Monograph (MORGAM) Study. *Stroke. 2011 Oct;42(10):2872-2877.*

[20] American College of Sports Medicine Position Stand. The recommended quantity and quality of exercise for developing and maintaining cardiorespiratory and muscular fitness, and flexibility in healthy adults. *Med Sci Sports Exerc. 1998 Jun;30(6):975-91. Review.*

[21] Schöpper H, Palme R, Ruf T, Huber S. Chronic stress in pregnant guinea pigs(Cavia aperea f. porcellus) attenuates long-term stress hormone levels and body weight gain, but not reproductive output. *J Comp Physiol B. 2011 Jun 7.*

[22] Wright YL. *Secrets about Bioidentical Hormones to Lose Fat and Prevent Cancer, Heart Disease, Menopause, and Andropause, by Optimizing Adrenals, Thyroid, Estrogen, Progesterone, Testosterone, and Growth Hormone!* Lulu.com. 2010. p 35.

[23] Wright, YL. *Secrets About Growth Hormone to Build Muscle, Increase Bone Density, and Burn Body Fat!* Lulu.com. 2011.

[24] Saleh Y, El-Oteify M, Abd-El-Salam AE, Tohamy A, Abd-Elsayed AA. Safety and benefits of large-volume liposuction: a single center experience. *Int Arch Med. 2009 Feb 2;2(1):4.*

[25] Vogt T, Belluscio D. Controversies in plastic surgery: suction-assisted lipectomy (SAL) and the hCG (human chorionic gonadotropin) protocol for obesity treatment. *Aesthetic Plast Surg. 1987;11(3):131-56. Review.*

[26] Ben-David K, Rossidis G. Bariatric surgery: indications, safety and efficacy. *Curr Pharm Des. 2011;17(12):1209-17. Review.*

[27] Padwal R, Klarenbach S, Wiebe N, Hazel M, Birch D, Karmali S, Sharma AM, Manns B, Tonelli M. Bariatric surgery: a systematic review of the clinical and economic evidence. *J Gen Intern Med. 2011 Oct;26(10):1183-94.*

[28] Kim DS, Kim TW, Park IK, Kang JS, Om AS. Effects of chromium picolinate supplementation on insulin sensitivity, serum lipids, and body weight in dexamethasone-treated rats. *Metabolism. 2002 May;51(5):589-94.*

[29] Farah A, Monteiro M, Donangelo CM, Lafay S. Chlorogenic acids from green coffee extract are highly bioavailable in humans. *J Nutr. 2008 Dec;138(12):2309-15.*

[30] Barrett ML, Udani JK. A proprietary alpha-amylase inhibitor from white bean (Phaseolus vulgaris): a review of clinical studies on weight loss and glycemic control. *Nutr J. 2011 Mar 17;10:24. Review.*

[31] Preuss HG, Rao CV, Garis R, Bramble JD, Ohia SE, Bagchi M, Bagchi D. An overview of the safety and efficacy of a novel, natural(-)-hydroxycitric acidextract (HCA-SX) for weight management. *J Med. 2004;35(1-6):33-48.*

[32] Nagao T, Komine Y, Soga S, Meguro S, Hase T, Tanaka Y, Tokimitsu I. Ingestion of a tea rich in catechins leads to a reduction in body fat and malondialdehyde-modified LDL in men. *Am J Clin Nutr. 2005 Jan;81(1):122-9.*

[33] Bolkent S, Bolkent S, Yanardag R, Tunali S. Protective effect of vanadyl sulfate on the pancreas of streptozotocin-induced diabetic rats. *Diabetes Res Clin Pract. 2005 Nov;70(2):103-9.*

[34] Trayhurn P. The biology of obesity. *Proc Nutr Soc. 2005 Feb;64(1):31-8.*

[35] Ngondi JL, Oben JE, Minka SR. The effect of Irvingia gabonensis seeds on body weight and blood lipids of obese subjects in Cameroon. *Lipids Health Dis. 2005 May 25;4:12.*

[36] Sahu A. Leptin signaling in the hypothalamus: emphasis on energy homeostasis and leptin resistance. *Front Neuroendocrinol. 2003 Dec;24(4):225-53.*

[37] Bell C, Abrams J, Nutt D. Tryptophan depletion and its implications for psychiatry. *Br J Psychiatry. 2001 May;178:399-405.*

[38] Wurtman RJ, Wurtman JJ. Brain Serotonin, Carbohydrate-craving, obesity and depression. *Adv Exp Med Biol. 1996;398:35-41.*

[39] Gendall, KA. Joyce, PR. Meal-induced changes in tryptophan: LNAA ratio: effects on craving and binge eating. *Eat Behav. 2000 Sep; 1(1):53-62.*

[40] Wellman NS, Friedberg B. Causes and consequences of adult obesity: health, social and

60   Fat Loss Secrets that Really Work!

economic impacts in the United States. *Asia Pac J Clin Nutr. 2002 Dec;11 Suppl 8:S705-9.*

[41] Wilson JH, Lamberts SW. The effect of triiodothyronine on weight loss and nitrogen balance of obese patients on a very-low-calorie liquid-formula diet. *Int J Obes. 1981;5(3):279-82.*

[42] Andersen RE, Wadden TA, Herzog RJ. Changes in bone mineral content in obese dieting women. *Metabolism. 1997 Aug;46(8):857-61.*

[43] Kamrath RO, Plummer LJ, Sadur CN, Adler MA, Strader WJ, Young RL, Weinstein RL. Cholelithiasis in patients treated with a very-low-calorie diet. *Am J Clin Nutr. 1992 Jul;56(1 Suppl):255S-257S.*

[44] Arai K, Miura J, Ohno M, Yokoyama J, Ikeda Y. Comparison of clinical usefulness of very-low-calorie diet and supplemental low-calorie diet. *Am J Clin Nutr. 1992 Jul;56(1 Suppl):275S-276S.*

[45] Wright YL. *Secrets about the HCG Diet! Treatment Guide, Controversy, Benefits, Risks, Side Effects, and Contraindications.* Lulu.com. 2011.

[46] Nettleton JA, Lutsey PL, Wang Y, Lima JA, Michos ED, Jacobs DR Jr. Diet soda intake and risk of incident metabolic syndrome and type 2 diabetes in the Multi-Ethnic Study of Atherosclerosis (MESA*). Diabetes Care. 2009 Apr;32(4):688-94.*

[47] Cantin L, Lenoir M, Augier E, Vanhille N, Dubreucq S, Serre F, Vouillac C,Ahmed SH. Cocaine is low on the value ladder of rats: possible evidence for resilience to addiction. *PLoS One. 2010 Jul 28;5(7):e11592.*

[48] Wright YL. *Secrets about Bioidentical Hormones to Lose Fat and Prevent Cancer, Heart Disease, Menopause, and Andropause, by Optimizing Adrenals, Thyroid, Estrogen, Progesterone, Testosterone, and Growth Hormone!* Lulu.com. 2010.

[49] Nettleton JA, Lutsey PL, Wang Y, Lima JA, Michos ED, Jacobs DR Jr. Diet soda intake and risk of incident metabolic syndrome and type 2 diabetes in the Multi-Ethnic Study of Atherosclerosis (MESA). *Diabetes Care. 2009 Apr;32(4):688-94.*

[50] Brown CM, Dulloo AG, Montani JP. Sugary drinks in the pathogenesis of obesity and cardiovascular diseases. *Int J Obes (Lond). 2008 Dec;32 Suppl 6:S28-34. Review.*

[51] Stanhope KL. Role of Fructose-Containing Sugars in the Epidemics of Obesity and Metabolic Syndrome. *Annu Rev Med. 2011 Jan 26.*

[52] Mostafalou S, Eghbal MA, Nili-Ahmadabadi A, Baeeri M, Abdollahi M. Biochemical evidence on the potential role of organophosphates in hepatic glucose metabolism toward insulin resistance through inflammatory signaling and free radical pathways. *Toxicol Ind Health. 2011 Nov 14.*

[53] Okosun IS, Liao Y, Rotimi CN, Prewitt TE, Cooper RS. Abdominal adiposity and clustering of multiple metabolic syndrome in White, Black and Hispanic americans. *Ann Epidemiol. 2000 Jul;10(5):263-70.*

[54] Hevener AL, Febbraio MA; Stock Conference Working Group. The 2009 stock conference report: inflammation, obesity and metabolic disease. *Obes Rev. 2010 Sep;11(9):635-44.*

[55] Després JP, Lemieux I. Abdominal obesity and metabolic syndrome. *Nature. 2006 Dec 14;444(7121):881-7. Review.*

[56] Haffner SM. Abdominal adiposity and cardiometabolic risk: do we have all the answers? *Am J Med. 2007 Sep;120(9 Suppl 1):S10-6; discussion S16-7. Review.*

[57] Hillon P, Guiu B, Vincent J, Petit JM. Obesity, type 2 diabetes and risk of digestive cancer. *Gastroenterol Clin Biol. 2010 Oct;34(10):529-33.*

[58] Hauner H. [Abdominal obesity and coronary heart disease. Pathophysiology and clinical significance]. *Herz. 1995 Feb;20(1):47-55. Review. German.*

[59] Harrell JS, Jessup A, Greene N. Changing our future: obesity and the metabolic syndrome in children and adolescents. *J Cardiovasc Nurs. 2006 Jul-Aug;21(4):322-30.*

[60] Reducing sugary beverage consumption in childhood may lessen chronic disease risk. *J Am Dent Assoc. 2007 Feb;138(2):160.*

[61] LaManna JC, Salem N, Puchowicz M, Erokwu B, Koppaka S, Flask C, Lee Z. Ketones suppress brain glucose consumption. *Adv Exp Med Biol. 2009;645:301-6.*

[62] www.metametrix.com

[63] http://www.metametrixinstitute.org/post/2009/06/17/Which-Test-to-Run.aspx

[64] Nakagawa Y, Nagasawa M, Yamada S, Hara A, Mogami H, Nikolaev VO, Lohse MJ, Shigemura N, Ninomiya Y, Kojima I. Sweet taste receptor expressed in pancreatic beta-cells activates the calcium and cyclic AMP signaling systems and stimulates insulin secretion. *PLoS One. 2009;4(4):e5106.*

[65] Ellingboe J. Acute effects of ethanol on sex hormones in non-alcoholic men and women. *Alcohol Alcohol Suppl. 1987;1:109-16.*

[66] Boyden TW, Silvert MA, Pamenter RW. Chronic ethanol feeding impairs human chorionic gonadotropin-stimulated testicular testosterone responses of dogs. *Biol Reprod. 1982 Oct;27(3):652-7.*

[67] Onland-Moret NC, Peeters PH, van der Schouw YT, Grobbee DE, van Gils CH. Alcohol and endogenous sex steroid levels in postmenopausal women: a cross-sectional study. *J Clin Endocrinol Metab. 2005 Mar;90(3):1414-9.*

[68] Schatzkin A, Longnecker MP. Alcohol and breast cancer. Where are we now and where do we go from here? *Cancer. 1994 Aug 1;74(3 Suppl):1101-10. Review.*

[69] Hakim RB, Gray RH, Zacur H. Alcohol and caffeine consumption and decreased fertility. *Fertil Steril. 1998 Oct;70(4):632-7.*

[70] García-Valdecasas-Campelo E, González-Reimers E, Santolaria-Fernández F, De La Vega-Prieto MJ, Milena-Abril A, Sánchez-Pérez MJ, Martínez-Riera A, Rodríguez-Rodríguez E. Brain atrophy in alcoholics: relationship with alcohol intake; liver disease; nutritional status, and inflammation. *Alcohol. 2007 Nov-Dec;42(6):533-8.*

[71] Vary TC, Frost RA, Lang CH. Acute alcohol intoxication increases atrogin-1 and MuRF1 mRNA without increasing proteolysis in skeletal muscle. *Am J Physiol Regul Integr Comp Physiol. 2008 Jun;294(6):R1777-89.*

[72] Barbosa JC, Shultz TD, Filley SJ, Nieman DC. The relationship among adiposity, diet, and hormone concentrations in vegetarian and nonvegetarian postmenopausal women. *Am J Clin Nutr. 1990 May;51(5):798-803.*

[73] Lee H, Wang Q, Yang F, Tao P, Li H, Huang Y, Li JY. SULT1A1 Arg213His Polymorphism, Smoked Meat, and Breast Cancer Risk: A Case-Control Study and Meta-Analysis. *DNA Cell Biol. 2011 Oct 19.*

[74] Heller RF, Hartley RM, Lewis B. The effect on blood lipids of eating charcoal-grilled meat. *Atherosclerosis. 1983 Aug;48(2):185-92.*

[75] Panesar NS, Chan KW. Decreased steroid hormone synthesis from inorganic nitrite and nitrate: studies in vitro and in vivo. *Toxicol Appl Pharmacol. 2000 Dec 15;169(3):222-30.*

[76] Cappon JP, Ipp E, Brasel JA, Cooper DM. Acute effects of high fat and high glucose meals on the growth hormone response to exercise. *J Clin Endocrinol Metab. 1993 Jun;76(6):1418-22.*

[77] de Koning L, Fung TT, Liao X, Chiuve SE, Rimm EB, Willett WC, Spiegelman D, Hu FB. Low-carbohydrate diet scores and risk of type 2 diabetes in men. *Am J Clin Nutr. 2011 Apr;93(4):844-50.*

[78] Wang C, Catlin DH, Starcevic B, Heber D, Ambler C, Berman N, Lucas G, Leung A, Schramm K, Lee PW, Hull L, Swerdloff RS. Low-fat high-fiber diet decreased serum and urine androgens in men. *J Clin Endocrinol Metab. 2005 Jun;90(6):3550-9.*

[79] Goldin BR, Woods MN, Spiegelman DL, Longcope C, Morrill-LaBrode A, Dwyer JT,Gualtieri LJ, Hertzmark E, Gorbach SL. The effect of dietary fat and fiber on serum estrogen concentrations in premenopausal women under controlled dietary conditions. *Cancer. 1994 Aug 1;74(3 Suppl):1125-31.*

[80] Ingram DM, Bennett FC, Willcox D, de Klerk N. Effect of low-fat diet on female sex hormone levels. *J Natl Cancer Inst. 1987 Dec;79(6):1225-9.*

[81] Braddock M. 11th annual Inflammatory and Immune Diseases Drug Discovery and Development Summit 12-13 March 2007, San Francisco, USA. *Expert Opin Investig Drugs. 2007 Jun;16(6):909-17.*

[82] Bendsen NT, Haugaard SB, Larsen TM, Chabanova E, Stender S, Astrup A. Effect of trans-fatty acid intake on insulin sensitivity and intramuscular lipids—a randomized trial in overweight postmenopausal women. *Metabolism. 2011 Jul;60(7):906-13.*

[83] Miller JK, Swanson EW, Lyke WA, Byrne WF. Altering iodine metabolism in the calf by feeding iodine-binding agents. *J Dairy Sci. 1975 Jun;58(6):931-7.*

[84] Eremin IuN, Kalinina NI. [Character of the changes in the thyroid gland of animals maintained on a vegetable oil diet]. *Vopr Pitan. 1977 Nov-Dec;(6):55-8. Russian.*

[85] Remig V, Franklin B, Margolis S, Kostas G, Nece T, Street JC. Trans fats in America: a review of their use, consumption, health implications, and regulation. *J Am Diet Assoc. 2010 Apr;110(4):585-92. Review.*

[86] Okuyama H, Ohara N, Tatematsu K, Fuma S, Nonogaki T, Yamada K, Ichikawa Y, Miyazawa D, Yasui Y, Honma S. Testosterone-lowering activity of canola and hydrogenated soybean oil in the stroke-prone spontaneously hypertensive rat. *JToxicol Sci. 2010 Oct;35(5):743-7.*

[87] Schlienger JL, Luca F, Vinzio S, Pradignac A. [Obesity and cancer]. *Rev Med Interne. 2009 Sep;30(9):776-82 Review. French.*

[88] Vahl N, Jørgensen JO, Skjaerbaek C, Veldhuis JD, Orskov H, Christiansen JS. Abdominal adiposity rather than age and sex predicts mass and regularity of GH secretion in healthy adults. *Am J Physiol. 1997 Jun;272(6 Pt 1):E1108-16.*

[89] Couillard C, Ruel G, Archer WR, Pomerleau S, Bergeron J, Couture P, Lamarche B, Bergeron N. Circulating levels of oxidative stress markers and endothelial adhesion molecules in men with abdominal obesity. *J Clin Endocrinol Metab. 2005 Dec;90(12):6454-9.*

[90] Charles LE, Burchfiel CM, Violanti JM, Fekedulegn D, Slaven JE, Browne RW, Hartley TA, Andrew ME. Adiposity measures and oxidative stress among police officers. *Obesity (Silver Spring). 2008 Nov;16(11):2489-97.*

[91] Mahoney CP. Adolescent gynecomastia. Differential diagnosis and management. *Pediatr Clin North Am. 1990 Dec;37(6):1389-404. Review.*

[92] Yu S, Zhang Y, Yuen MT, Zou C, Danielpour D, Chan FL. 17-Beta-estradiol induces neoplastic transformation in prostatic epithelial cells. *Cancer Lett.2011 May 1;304(1):8-20.*

[93] Nicklas BJ, Cesari M, Penninx BW, Kritchevsky SB, Ding J, Newman A, Kitzman DW, Kanaya AM, Pahor M, Harris TB. Abdominal obesity is an independent risk factor for chronic heart failure in older people. *J Am Geriatr Soc. 2006 Mar;54(3):413-20.*

[94] Wright YL. *Secrets about Bioidentical Hormones to Lose Fat and Prevent Cancer, Heart Disease, Menopause, and Andropause, by Optimizing Adrenals, Thyroid, Estrogen, Progesterone, Testosterone, and Growth Hormone!* Lulu.com. 2010.

[95] Wright YL. *Bioidentical Hormones Made Easy!* Lulu.com. 2011

[96] Wright YL. *Secrets about Growth Hormone To Build Muscle Mass, Increase Bone Density, And Burn Body Fat!* Lulu.com. 2011

[97] Wright YL. *Secrets about Bioidentical Hormones to Lose Fat and Prevent Cancer, Heart Disease, Menopause, and Andropause, by Optimizing Adrenals, Thyroid, Estrogen, Progesterone, Testosterone, and Growth Hormone!* Lulu.com. 2010. p 66.

[98] Wright YL. *Secrets about Bioidentical Hormones to Lose Fat and Prevent Cancer, Heart Disease, Menopause, and Andropause, by Optimizing Adrenals, Thyroid, Estrogen, Progesterone, Testosterone, and Growth Hormone!* Lulu.com. 2010. p 17.

[99] Travison TG, Araujo AB, O'Donnell AB, Kupelian V, McKinlay JB. A population-level decline in serum testosterone levels in American men. *J Clin Endocrinol Metab. 2007 Jan;92(1):196-202.*

[100] Hyde Z, Norman PE, Flicker L, Hankey GJ, Almeida OP, McCaul KA, Chubb SA, Yeap BB. Low Free Testosterone Predicts Mortality from Cardiovascular Disease But Not Other Causes: The Health in Men Study. *J Clin Endocrinol Metab. 2011 Oct 19.*

[101] Szymczak J, Milewicz A, Thijssen JH, Blankenstein MA, Daroszewski J. Concentration of sex steroids in adipose tissue after menopause. *Steroids. 1998 May-Jun;63(5-6):319-21.*

Fat Loss Secrets that Really Work! 63

[102] McTiernan A, Rajan KB, Tworoger SS, Irwin M, Bernstein L, Baumgartner R, Gilliland F, Stanczyk FZ, Yasui Y, Ballard-Barbash R. Adiposity and sex hormones in postmenopausal breast cancer survivors. *J Clin Oncol. 2003 May 15;21(10):1961-6.*

[103] Rossouw JE, Anderson GL, Prentice RL, LaCroix AZ, Kooperberg C, Stefanick ML, Jackson RD, Beresford SA, Howard BV, Johnson KC, Kotchen JM, Ockene J; Writing Group for the Women's Health Initiative Investigators. Risks and benefits of estrogen plus progestin in healthy postmenopausal women: principal results from the Women's Health Initiative randomized controlled trial. *JAMA. 2002 Jul 17;288(3):321-33.*

[104] Nesaretnam K, Corcoran D, Dils RR, Darbre P. 3,4,3',4'-Tetrachlorobiphenyl acts as an estrogen in vitro and in vivo. *Mol Endocrinol. 1996 Aug;10(8):923-36.*

[105] Spink DC, Lincoln DW 2nd, Dickerman HW, Gierthy JF. 2,3,7,8-Tetrachlorodibenzo-p-dioxin causes an extensive alteration of 17 beta-estradiol metabolism in MCF-7 breast tumor cells. *Proc Natl Acad Sci U S A. 1990 Sep;87(17):6917-21.*

[106] Wright YL. *Secrets about Bioidentical Hormones to Lose Fat and Prevent Cancer, Heart Disease, Menopause, and Andropause, by Optimizing Adrenals, Thyroid, Estrogen, Progesterone, Testosterone, and Growth Hormone!* Lulu.com. 2010. p 27.

[107] Wright YL. *Secrets about Bioidentical Hormones to Lose Fat and Prevent Cancer, Heart Disease, Menopause, and Andropause, by Optimizing Adrenals, Thyroid, Estrogen, Progesterone, Testosterone, and Growth Hormone!* Lulu.com. 2010. p 26.

[108] Roy JR, Chakraborty S, Chakraborty TR. Estrogen-like endocrine disrupting chemicals affecting puberty in humans--a review. *Med Sci Monit. 2009 Jun;15(6):RA137-45. Review.*

[109] Wright YL. *Secrets about Bioidentical Hormones to Lose Fat and Prevent Cancer, Heart Disease, Menopause, and Andropause, by Optimizing Adrenals, Thyroid, Estrogen, Progesterone, Testosterone, and Growth Hormone!* Lulu.com. 2010.

[110] Wright YL. *Bioidentical Hormones Made Easy!* Lulu.com. 2011

[111] Wright YL. *Secrets about Growth Hormone To Build Muscle Mass, Increase Bone Density, And Burn Body Fat!* Lulu.com. 2011

[112] Ordóñez P, Moreno M, Alonso A, Llaneza P, Díaz F, González C. 17beta-Estradiol and/or progesterone protect from insulin resistance in STZ-induced diabetic rats. *J Steroid Biochem Mol Biol. 2008 Sep;111(3-5):287-94.*

[113] Wright YL. *Secrets about Bioidentical Hormones to Lose Fat and Prevent Cancer, Heart Disease, Menopause, and Andropause, by Optimizing Adrenals, Thyroid, Estrogen, Progesterone, Testosterone, and Growth Hormone!* Lulu.com. 2010. p 28.

[114] Heerdt AS, Young CW, Borgen PI. Calcium glucarate as a chemopreventive agent in breast cancer. *Altern Med Rev. 2002 Aug; 7(4):336-9.*

[115] Wright YL. *Secrets about Bioidentical Hormones to Lose Fat and Prevent Cancer, Heart Disease, Menopause, and Andropause, by Optimizing Adrenals, Thyroid, Estrogen, Progesterone, Testosterone, and Growth Hormone!* Lulu.com. 2010. p 40.

[116] Wright YL. *Secrets about Bioidentical Hormones to Lose Fat and Prevent Cancer, Heart Disease, Menopause, and Andropause, by Optimizing Adrenals, Thyroid, Estrogen, Progesterone, Testosterone, and Growth Hormone!* Lulu.com. 2010. p 40.

[117] Wright YL. *Secrets about Bioidentical Hormones to Lose Fat and Prevent Cancer, Heart Disease, Menopause, and Andropause, by Optimizing Adrenals, Thyroid, Estrogen, Progesterone, Testosterone, and Growth Hormone!* Lulu.com. 2010. p 44.

[118] Pérez-de-Heredia F, Sánchez J, Priego T, Nicolás F, Portillo Mdel P, Palou A, Zamora S, Garaulet M. Adiponectin is involved in the protective effect of DHEA against metabolic risk in aged rats. *Steroids. 2008 Oct;73(11):1128-36.*

[119] Carter WJ, Faas FH, Perry CA, Lynch ME. Comparison of the effect of a protein-free and restricted high protein-low carbohydrate diet on ventricular myosin ATPase activity and isomyosin profile in young rats: evidence that protein-depleted animals are euthyroid. *J Nutr. 1987 Dec;117(12):2142-6.*

[120] Serog P, Apfelbaum M, Autissier N, Baigts F, Brigant L, Ktorza A. Effects of slimming and composition of diets on VO2 and thyroid hormones in healthy subjects. *Am J Clin Nutr.*

1982 Jan;35(1):24-35.
[121] Wright YL. *Secrets about Bioidentical Hormones to Lose Fat and Prevent Cancer, Heart Disease, Menopause, and Andropause, by Optimizing Adrenals, Thyroid, Estrogen, Progesterone, Testosterone, and Growth Hormone!* Lulu.com. 2010. p 51.
[122] Wilson JH, Lamberts SW. The effect of triiodothyronine on weight loss and nitrogen balance of obese patients on a very-low-calorie liquid-formula diet. *Int J Obes. 1981;5(3):279-82.*
[123] Morillo E, Gardner LI. Activation of latent Graves' disease in children. Review of possible psychosomatic mechanisms. *Clin Pediatr (Phila). 1980 Mar;19(3):160-3.*
[124] Torpy DJ, Tsigos C, Lotsikas AJ, Defensor R, Chrousos GP, Papanicolaou DA. Acute and delayed effects of a single-dose injection of interleukin-6 on thyroid function in healthy humans. *Metabolism. 1998 Oct;47(10):1289-93.*
[125] Wright YL. *Secrets about Bioidentical Hormones to Lose Fat and Prevent Cancer, Heart Disease, Menopause, and Andropause, by Optimizing Adrenals, Thyroid, Estrogen, Progesterone, Testosterone, and Growth Hormone!* Lulu.com. 2010. p 53.
[126] Pearce EN. Thyroid dysfunction in perimenopausal and postmenopausal women. *Menopause Int. 2007 Mar;13(1):8-13. Review.*
[127] http://www.worldhealth.net/pages/directory/ 888-997-0112
[128] http://www.acamnet.org/ 800-532-3688
[129] Wright YL. *Secrets about Bioidentical Hormones to Lose Fat and Prevent Cancer, Heart Disease, Menopause, and Andropause, by Optimizing Adrenals, Thyroid, Estrogen, Progesterone, Testosterone, and Growth Hormone!* Lulu.com. 2010. p.78.
[130] Wright YL. *Secrets about Bioidentical Hormones to Lose Fat and Prevent Cancer, Heart Disease, Menopause, and Andropause, by Optimizing Adrenals, Thyroid, Estrogen, Progesterone, Testosterone, and Growth Hormone!* Lulu.com. 2010. p.27.
[131] Wright YL. *Secrets about Bioidentical Hormones to Lose Fat and Prevent Cancer, Heart Disease, Menopause, and Andropause, by Optimizing Adrenals, Thyroid, Estrogen, Progesterone, Testosterone, and Growth Hormone!* Lulu.com. 2010.

Printed in Great Britain
by Amazon.co.uk, Ltd.,
Marston Gate.